W9-ADD-457

The EVERYTHING Wedding Workout Book

Dear Reader,

Congratulations! I'm so happy for you as you undertake the planning for one of the most memorable occasions in your life. I know that you want to look and feel your absolute best—and I know that you will. Every bride is beautiful, and when it is your time to get married, you too will radiate the love, hope, and promise that you feel inside.

This book gives you the information that you need to get in shape for the big day. Regardless of your level of fitness, if you follow the step-by-step guidance set forth in these chapters, you'll be stronger, toned, and more healthy. You'll manage your stress better, enjoy deeper sleep, and have some fun time for yourself as well. You'll improve your nutrition and learn more about how to create a wellness lifestyle that will continue to serve you and your spouse long after your wedding day.

Use the information and workouts in this book to help you feel better about yourself; to learn how to have more energy; and to find even deeper ways to relax, let go, and recharge. Do the best that you can and applaud yourself for all your efforts. Every step in a positive direction counts!

Feel free to contact me via my Web site (*www.shirleyarcher.com*). I always appreciate hearing from my readers. I wish you much happiness and joy in creating your new wellness lifestyle. Thank you for inviting me to support you during this exciting time.

Sincere best wishes,

Shirley Archer

The EVERYTHING® Series

Editorial

Publishing Director	Gary M. Krebs
Director of Product Development	Paula Munier
Associate Managing Editor	Laura M. Daly
Associate Copy Chief	Brett Palana-Shanahan
Acquisitions Editor	Kate Burgo
Development Editor	Rachel Engelson
Associate Production Editor	Casey Ebert

Production

Director of Manufacturing	Susan Beale
Associate Director of Production	Michelle Roy Kelly
Cover Design	Paul Beatrice Matt LeBlanc Erick DaCosta
Design and Layout	Heather Barrett Brewster Brownville Colleen Cunningham Jennifer Oliveira
Series Cover Artist	Barry Littmann
Interior Illustrator	Eric Andrews

Visit the entire Everything® Series at *www.everything.com*

THE
EVERYTHING®
WEDDING
WORKOUT
BOOK

Look and feel your best for the big day

Shirley Archer

with Andrea Mattei,
author of *The "I Have a Life" Bride's Guide*

Adams Media
Avon, Massachusetts

*This book is dedicated to those who are beginning a new life together
with the one they love. Celebrate your wedding by putting your best
self forward and radiating your beauty from within.*

An Everything® Series Book.
Everything® and everything.com® are registered trademarks of F+W Publications, Inc.

Published by Adams Media, an F+W Publications Company
57 Littlefield Street, Avon, MA 02322 U.S.A.
www.adamsmedia.com

ISBN 10: 1-59337-721-5
ISBN 13: 978-1-59337-721-2

Printed in the United States of America.

J   I   H   G   F   E   D   C   B   A

Library of Congress Cataloging-in-Publication Data
Archer, Shirley.
The everything wedding workout book / Shirley Archer with Andrea Mattei.
p.   cm.
Includes index.
ISBN-13: 978-1-59337-721-2
ISBN-10: 1-59337-721-5
1. Exercise for women. 2. Brides--Health and hygiene. I. Mattei, Andrea. II. Title.
GV482.A73 2007
613.71082--dc22
2006028446

Disclaimer: The exercise program within The Everything® Wedding Workout Book or any other exercise program may result in injury. Consult your doctor before beginning this or any exercise program. If you begin to feel faint or dizzy while doing any of the exercises in this book, consult your doctor.

This publication is designed to provide accurate and authoritative information with regard to the subject matter covered. It is sold with the understanding that the publisher is not engaged in rendering legal, accounting, or other professional advice. If legal advice or other expert assistance is required, the services of a competent professional person should be sought.
—From a *Declaration of Principles* jointly adopted by a Committee of the American Bar Association and a Committee of Publishers and Associations

Many of the designations used by manufacturers and sellers to distinguish their products are claimed as trademarks. Where those designations appear in this book and Adams Media was aware of a trademark claim, the designations have been printed with initial capital letters.

*This book is available at quantity discounts for bulk purchases.
For information, please call 1-800-289-0963.*

Contents

Acknowledgments

Thanks to Marirose Charbonneau, Michael Pippitone at Power Music Productions, and Dudley and Dean Evenson at Soundings of the Planet for providing high-quality apparel and music. Particular kudos to Beverly Principal, Kay McGuire, and Zoran Popovic for photos. Much appreciation to Lauren Schoenthaler, Noel Hirst, Susan Swetter, Suzanne Serpas, and Dee White for valuable comments. Big hugs and gratitude to my dear sister Georgia Archer and to Anthony Dominici for their love and support always. Very special acknowledgment to René Eichenberger for his unique inspiration and motivation in seeing me through to the last word.

Top Ten Ways to Get in Shape
for Your Wedding Day

1. Do your best each day to move more—park farther away, use stairs, and walk to run errands.

2. Avoid doing too much activity too soon. Increase your training slowly and steadily to avoid injuries.

3. Balance your program with walking, strength and toning moves, stretches, mind-body exercises, and deep breathing.

4. Use your workout time as a way to release stress and take care of yourself, not as another stressful item on your to-do list.

5. Tell everyone about your shape-up goals and get the support of your friends, family, and fiancé to be more active, eat properly, and manage stress.

6. Visualize yourself at a healthy weight and in your ideal shape. Train to be the best you, not to look like a supermodel.

7. Set realistic goals, track your progress, and congratulate yourself for all your positive achievements.

8. Don't beat yourself up or engage in negative self-talk if you get too busy and don't stick to your planned routine. Simply start fresh the next day.

9. Do something active daily. Squeeze in squats, lunges, pushups, and other exercises throughout your day if you can't make it to the gym.

10. Walk as much as possible with friends, co-workers, family, or even a friendly dog to manage weight, relieve stress, and stay fit.

Introduction

▶ You're ready to embark on a journey of a lifetime as you prepare for one of the happiest days of your life. All eyes will be on you for the series of social events—the important and timeless rituals—that mark this momentous occasion. You want to look and feel your absolute best among your dearest friends and family members.

During this pre-wedding planning period, *The Everything® Wedding Workout Book* is your comprehensive guide to achieving your fitness and wellness goals. Step by step, the information in this book helps you to become a radiant, picture-perfect bride on your wedding day.

You have enough on your plate. Don't waste precious time trying to guess what's the best way to slim down and tone up for your memorable day. Lean on professionals for informed advice. Training for your wedding is like training for an important athletic event—an experienced coach helps. The date is fixed. The countdown is on. Your time is limited, every workout counts, and for the best outcome, you simply cannot wait until the last minute. You can start now with the support and information contained within these pages.

The most useful programs have both structure and flexibility. This handbook provides up-to-date, practical, professional advice on how to mentally prepare for your wedding shape-up program; how to establish long- and short-term goals; how to integrate cardio and weight training, stretching, and mind-body exercise like yoga and Pilates for a strong and healthy mind and body; how to include relaxation and stress management in your jam-packed schedule to cultivate a calm and peaceful spirit; how to make intelligent, healthy eating choices for successful weight management and optimal well-being; and, how to cope with temporary setbacks and obstacles with ease and grace. Basically, if it's part of a wellness program for you to look, feel, and be your best on your wedding day, it's included in this book.

Before you set your training program in motion, you need to know your starting point. This book begins with a series of assessments to evaluate your current levels of fitness and wellness. Then, your program is targeted to address areas where you need the most work. This program is realistic and filled with proven holistic strategies on how to increase your lifestyle activity for more fitness benefits; how to recruit support from your fiancé, family, and friends; and even how to incorporate your pet into your training program for best results.

Looking your best in your wedding gown requires particular attention to a few certain essential areas. Most wedding dresses show off your arms, shoulders, the décolleté, and back and all require good posture for the best presentation. In addition to your face and hair, these parts of your physique are also the most featured in photographic memories that will be preserved for the ages. *The Everything*® *Wedding Workout Book* includes toning and stretching exercises that address these specific areas. If you follow all the instructions, you will shine with confidence and happiness on your wedding day.

The only remaining ingredient is you. Consistency is key to your success. Even if you stray from your program, you can get right back to it. Besides, the more progress you make, the more fine-tuning you can do in the final weeks as the special date approaches. All the workouts in this book are targeted to bringing out your best for a peak presentation on your most important day. In fact, you may find that you feel so great and receive so many compliments that you'll be inspired to keep up all the great work long after the wedding day passes. Start now by seeing yourself walk down the wedding aisle, confidently putting your best self forward.

Chapter 1

Congratulations, You're Engaged!

You're ready to become your most radiant and healthy self, excited to dazzle everyone on your special day. Before you begin your training and wellness program, you must understand some basic concepts and know your starting point. In this chapter, you will review training principles to help you understand why your program has a variety of components. You will also evaluate your current fitness level so you know what to work on. You will also learn how your current nutrition, relaxation, and sleep habits contribute to your overall well-being.

Getting in Your Top Shape

Taking that first step with a new shape-up program is always challenging, yet also exciting. Think of it as starting a training adventure that will peak during some of the most memorable moments of your life. If you have the commitment to get married, you can harness your spirit of commitment to get in your best shape ever. As in any relationship, your positive attitude about yourself will help you through many challenges. However, finding the right program for you is just as important as your dedication.

Know Before You Start

Brides are beautiful because they glow from within, reflecting the love and joy that they feel. As you prepare for your important day, keep perspective on why you're training and what your training will do for you. Radiance from within is really the result of optimal health and well-being from taking good care of yourself in mind, body, and spirit. You're training to be the best you—not to look like a supermodel or a celebrity—but to embrace your best self. To achieve this goal, you need to consider what it means. True wellness includes physical, mental, emotional, social, and spiritual dimensions. These components are all interrelated.

Components of Wellness

The components of wellness include the following:

- **Physical wellness**—The health of your body is affected by whether you maintain minimal levels of physical fitness, whether you eat nutritious foods, and whether you restore your body with quality rest. It is negatively affected by harmful habits such as smoking, overeating junk foods, or excessive consumption of alcohol.
- **Mental wellness**—Mental health refers to the strength of your reasoning abilities and cognitive skills—whether you are able to learn, understand information, and apply knowledge.
- **Emotional wellness**—Emotional well-being consists of feeling good about who you are. A positive attitude in life contributes to

emotional wellness. Whether you effectively manage stress can negatively affect your mental, emotional, and physical well-being.

- **Social wellness**—Enjoying a strong network of friends and family, even a close relationship with a pet, is important to staying healthy, strengthening your immune system, and improving the quality and longevity of your life.

- **Spiritual wellness**—Spiritual beliefs, independent of physical needs of the body, are also an important component of well-being. Feelings of inner peace and harmony with yourself and the world around you contribute to your spiritual health.

The program in this book provides a holistic approach that primarily focuses on the physical aspect of your overall wellness, while including tips and information regarding how to enhance your health in other dimensions so that you can achieve total well-being. Creating total wellness is really a matter of adopting healthy habits that integrate each of these aspects for a balanced approach to living well and producing health, which will serve both you and your spouse well during the many years of your married life.

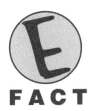

FACT

According to the Centers for Disease Control, about half of all deaths in the United States are related to behaviors that can be changed. Studies show that if you follow a way of life that promotes health, you can add as much as twenty years to your life. This is true even if you adopt healthy habits at the age of fifty.

Components of Fitness

Like wellness, fitness consists of a variety of elements that together create physical health. A broad definition of fitness is a state of well-being in which you have a low risk of developing health problems at a young age and you have plenty of energy to participate in a full, active lifestyle. Fitness is also achieved on a variety of levels. You can exercise to enjoy fitness for a healthy life or you can train to achieve the fitness of an Olympic athlete.

Neither approach is better than the other; it simply depends on your goals. The wedding workout program in this book focuses on fitness for health, which includes cardiovascular fitness; muscular strength; muscular endurance; flexibility; body composition; and balance, agility, and coordination.

Cardiovascular Fitness

Cardiovascular fitness is also called aerobic fitness or cardiovascular endurance, and refers to the condition of your heart and lungs. The more efficient your cardiorespiratory system is, the more able you are to use oxygen to create energy for continuous physical activity. If you have good cardiovascular fitness, this means that your heart is strong and conditioned and your lungs are healthy and efficient.

Muscular Strength

Muscular strength refers to the maximum amount of weight that you can lift at any one time—the force you can exert in one effort. This is also called your one-rep max. For example, if you can do only one squat while holding forty pounds of weight, that is your one rep max for the squat. Developing high levels of strength generally results in larger-sized muscles. Take a look at bodybuilders or power lifters for an idea of the results of working on muscular strength.

Muscular Endurance

Muscular endurance is the number of times you can lift a sub-maximal weight continuously over time without becoming tired. For example, if you can do twenty squats before your legs become too fatigued to do another one, that is how much endurance you have in your hip and thigh muscles. Developing a lot of muscular endurance typically results in leaner muscles. Take a look at the legs of marathon runners or karate experts.

Flexibility

Flexibility relates to your ability to move your joints fully and freely. For example, if the muscles in your lower back and in the backs of your legs are flexible, you can bend over and touch your toes. Flexibility is specific to each joint. For example, your hamstrings may be flexible but the muscles around your shoulders might still be tight. Maintaining flexibility gives you ease and grace in motion—perfect for gliding down the wedding aisle.

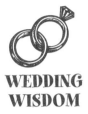

WEDDING WISDOM

It's easy to be sucked up into the constant barrage of details that fly your way when planning a wedding. Don't lose yourself in all those details. Remember: All wedding and no play make you a dull bride-to-be! Exercise is one way to take some much-needed time for yourself along that busy road to the altar.

Body Composition

Body composition is the term used to describe the components of your body that, when added up all together, make up your total body weight, meaning that it represents how much of your body is fat and how much of your body is not fat (muscles, bones, organs, and other vital tissues). Knowing your body composition is more valuable than knowing your weight. Body composition takes into account that some of us are larger-framed with bigger bones, whereas your weight does not. When you want to lose weight, you want to lose fat, not valuable lean muscle, and certainly not important bone density.

Balance, Agility, and Coordination

Balance, agility, and coordination are related to the neuromuscular system, in other words, the degree of effectiveness of the connection between your mind and your body. The more practice that you have executing moves that require balance, agility, and coordination on a progressive basis, the more you will improve these skill areas.

Poor balance is a leading contributor to falls in older adults, which can have fatal consequences. In the United States, one out of three adults over age sixty-five fall. Twenty-five percent of people over age fifty who fall and break a hip bone die within the first year following their hip fracture. Unless you actively practice, you begin to lose your balance skills starting around age thirty.

Principles of Fitness Training

To achieve fitness in all six components of fitness, a good training program includes four training principles. These are known by the acronym FITT:

- **Frequency**—This refers to how many days per week you need to do particular exercises.
- **Intensity**—This relates to how hard your body's working during exercise.
- **Time**—This principle concerns how long the exercise session lasts.
- **Type**—This refers to the kind of exercise activity.

For example, to get aerobically fit, you need to exercise at least four days a week, at 40 to 60 percent of your maximum heart rate, for at least thirty minutes, by doing a rhythmic activity that uses the large muscles of the lower body such as walking, jogging, swimming, or bicycling.

Seeing Results

To achieve good training results, progress your training gradually to avoid injury, incorporate the specificity principle so that you get the results that you want, and use the overload principle for optimal training gains. Specificity is an important principle of training. Your body adapts to the particular demands that you make. For example, if you want stronger legs, you need to do squats and lunges, not sit-ups. If you have a specific goal, such as toned shoulders and upper arms, you must train in a way that targets achieving that specific result. Overload simply means that if you want to get training results, you need to challenge your body—your heart, lungs, muscles, and nervous system—to the stresses of exercise at a level that is beyond what it's used to doing. By combining the variables of frequency, intensity, time, and type, you can progressively overload your body and improve fitness.

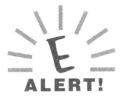

"Overload" might be the motto when it comes to creating a challenging exercise training program, but think twice when it comes to your wedding plans. Don't overwhelm yourself by trying to plan your entire wedding in a pinch. Especially if you're having a big wedding, set a realistic timeline and then stick to it!

Focusing only on fitness, however, does not achieve the result of radiant health and beauty. In addition to a good fitness training program, paying attention to good posture, nutrition, and rest and relaxation contributes to achieving the total well-being that gives you a healthy glow and helps you to enjoy life to its fullest. Committing to your well-being before embarking on your life together with your partner gives you both a strong foundation for creating a healthy and happy life as a couple.

Assessing Your Current Fitness Level

Simply put, assessments are tools to help you know yourself. When you know where you're starting from, it's much easier to plan an efficient route to your destination. Fitness appraisals provide you with data points so you have a record of your progress—think of them as snapshots of various stops along the way to your goal. Before you take any of the following fitness tests be sure to take the PAR-Q (Physical Activity Readiness Questionnaire) in Appendix A. For best results, repeat these tests no more than once every two months. Give yourself time to improve between tests. Record your results in Appendix B, Chart Your Progress.

Studies show that keeping a record of your activities can help you to achieve your goals and create lasting healthy habits. Each person is different. If you think that tracking your progress will motivate you to stick with your program, give it a try. Keep records on a daily, weekly, or monthly basis—whatever works best for your life. Be sure to reward yourself for meeting both short- and long-term goals.

MEASURE YOUR AEROBIC FITNESS

EQUIPMENT Stopwatch or watch. Wear a pedometer if you have one.

GET READY Find a local indoor or outdoor track where you can measure how far you walk. Most tracks are either one-fourth mile or 800 meters, which is approximately one-fourth mile.

ACTION Start your stopwatch or note the time on your watch and begin walking around the track from the starting line. If you're not using a stop watch, start at an easily remembered point such as on the hour, quarter hour, or half hour. Walk four laps around the track at a comfortable pace. Depending on your level of fitness, you can push yourself harder and walk at a brisk pace.

MEASUREMENTS When you cross the starting point of your fourth lap, click your stop watch or note the time on your watch. Record the number of steps on your pedometer. Record the amount of time in minutes and seconds that it took for you to walk four laps.

MEASURE YOUR UPPER BODY STRENGTH

EQUIPMENT Exercise mat, towel, or a comfortable carpeted surface.

GET READY Kneel on all fours on the floor. Walk your hands forward until your hands are slightly wider than shoulder width apart and your torso resembles a slanted board. Tighten your abdominal muscles by pulling your belly in toward your spine. Lengthen your torso; avoid arching your back. If you prefer, select another variation, depending on your current level of strength.

ACTION Do pushups by bending your elbows and lowering your torso toward the ground. Straighten your arms and push your body up through your palms. Keep your shoulders relaxed; avoid arching your back.

MEASUREMENTS Count as you perform as many pushups as you can with complete range of motion. When you can no longer maintain form, that repetition does not count. For example, if you start to arch your back and drop your belly toward the ground, it means that you can no longer maintain form and should stop. Record the number of pushups, as well as whether you did them against a wall, on your knees or toes, or in a slant board or tabletop position. When you repeat the test, be sure to use the same style.

TIPS Inhale to prepare, exhale as you push up. Inhale as you lower your torso as low as possible. In the elevated position, avoid locking your elbows. Keep your neck long and straight. Avoid dropping your head. If your wrists are uncomfortable, place a rolled towel under the palms of your hands while your fingers remain on the floor. This reduces the angle at the wrist joint and alleviates pressure.

Your wrists may be uncomfortable due to weak forearm muscles. Alternatives to placing a rolled towel under the palm include holding dumbbells in your hands to elevate your hands so you can keep the wrist joint straight, or doing exercises on your closed fists.

VARIATIONS

(EASIER) If it is not comfortable for you to kneel on the floor, you can do this exercise against a wall. Stand in front of a wall. Place palms on the wall slightly wider than shoulder width apart, directly under the shoulder line. Bend elbows and lower torso toward the wall. Straighten arms as you push through your hands.

(EASIER) On the floor, instead of working from a slant board position, kneel on all fours in a tabletop position. Lower your chest toward the floor by bending your elbows. Adjust the load by shifting more or less weight from your knees onto your hands. Put as much weight on your hands as you are able to tolerate and execute a pushup with correct form.

(HARDER) On the floor, instead of working from a slant board position, straighten your legs and rest on the balls of your feet, so your body resembles a plank.

MEASURE YOUR ABDOMINAL AND CORE FITNESS

EQUIPMENT Exercise mat, towel, or a comfortable carpeted surface and a wall clock or timer.

GET READY Lie on your back on the mat with your knees bent at a ninety-degree angle and your feet flat on the floor. Place the palms of your hands on your thighs. Tuck your chin in slightly, keeping a feeling of length in the back of your neck.

ACTION Set the timer for one minute. If you're not using a timer, watch a clock that you can easily see, or use a watch with a second hand. Start at the beginning of a minute, if you're using a second hand to measure time. Count each complete repetition as you slide your palms toward your knees as you curl your body up. Make sure that your fingertips reach the top of your knees before you curl back down. It helps if you count aloud.

MEASUREMENTS At the end of one minute, note how many sit-ups you completed. Record it on your progress chart.

TIPS Inhale to prepare, exhale as you curl up, and inhale as you roll down. This style of sit-up is not recommended for training purposes because it also uses muscles in your legs. It's useful, however, as a general measure of muscular endurance. Because it uses many hip flexors, it's really a measure of the endurance in both your abdominal and hip flexor muscles.

MEASURE YOUR FLEXIBILITY

EQUIPMENT An exercise mat, masking tape, and a yardstick.

GET READY Use the masking tape to attach the yardstick lengthwise in the center of the exercise mat right across the fifteen-inch mark. The masking tape should run cross-wise over the width of the mat and secure the yardstick in place. Take off your shoes. Sit on the mat with your legs stretched out in front of you in a straddle position. Place your heels on the edge of the tape right at the fifteen-inch marking.

ACTION Relax your shoulders. Place one hand on top of the other. Place the palm of the bottom hand on top of the yardstick. Take a nice deep breath. As you exhale, lean forward from your hips and slide the palm of your bottom hand forward on the mat along the yardstick.

MEASUREMENTS Make three attempts. Each time, note how far the farthest tip of your finger made it on the yardstick. Record the best score out of your three attempts on your progress chart.

TIPS Stay relaxed. If you feel tension on the tops of your thighs, go ahead and bend your knees slightly.

ANALYZE YOUR POSTURE

Good posture, also referred to as good alignment, not only looks great, but also prevents back pain, muscle aches, pinched nerves, and joint injuries. You can look up to five pounds slimmer and gain up to an inch in height simply by standing up properly. When your spine is aligned correctly, your ear, shoulder, hip, knee and ankle line up with each other vertically. The natural, gentle *S* shape of the spinal column is retained and your spinal discs are not excessively compressed.

A good training program leads to balanced muscle development and good alignment. Poor postural habits can lead to chronic muscular tension, headaches, restricted blood flow, pinched nerves, faulty breathing patterns, poor digestion, and reduced overall health and well-being. Good posture helps you to stand out in a crowd and reflects confidence and health—all wonderful attributes to help you shine on your wedding day.

Before you begin your wedding workout program, assess your posture to create a benchmark against which to measure your progress.

EQUIPMENT A full-length mirror, form-fitting clothing that enables you to see your physique, and a wall with a visible vertical line from floor to ceiling such as a corner, sliding glass door, or other design feature. If possible, it is ideal to have a friend or family member with a camera.

GET READY Stand naturally, facing sideways, in front of the full-length mirror. If you have a friend and a camera, stand sideways directly in front of a vertical line such as a corner of the room, or the edge of a sliding glass door so that the vertical line is parallel to the center of your body.

ACTION Have your friend take a picture. Paste the photo on your progress chart. Draw a vertical line down the center. If you can't take a photo, simply turn your head to view yourself in the mirror and check your alignment.

MEASUREMENTS Check the photo to see whether your ears and the midpoints of your shoulders, hips, knees, and ankles are in a straight line. Notice whether your lower back is flat, excessively arched, or has a relaxed, natural curve. Notice whether your palms face the sides of your body or your shoulders round forward with your palms facing back.

TIPS Your goal is to achieve good alignment along the vertical line with a level chin, relaxed shoulders, and your arms hanging at your sides with your palms facing in.

An excessive arch in the lower back usually means that your hip flexors are tight and that the muscles of your buttocks are weak. Sitting for long hours compresses the lower spine and leads to tightness in the thighs because your legs are bent at the hip. Get up frequently and stretch every hour if you have a job that requires you to sit for long periods of time.

Test Your Nutrition I.Q.

To be your best, you need to nourish your body with healthy foods. When you're juggling everything on your busy calendar preparing for your wedding, it may be challenging to eat properly. However, it is well worth your time to learn the principles of good nutrition and make an effort to make smart food choices and to exercise portion control.

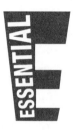

Resist the urge to crash diet during your wedding countdown. Good nutrition is an essential part of any healthy lifestyle, and you need enough energy to follow through with your wedding workouts. There's no "perfect" body—exercise and eat right to make the most of *your* assets. You want to look healthy on your wedding day, not stick thin!

Healthy eating is the foundation for feeling great, preventing diseases, and maintaining a strong body and a healthy weight. Evaluate your nutrition know-how by taking the following quiz.

Nutrition Quiz

1. What is the recommended daily amount of fruit consumption based on a 2,000-calorie diet? ....

2. What is the recommended daily amount of vegetable consumption based on a 2,000-calorie diet? ....

3. What are the five vegetable subgroups that you should eat several times each week?

    ....

    ....

4. How many ounces of whole-grain products are recommended as a daily minimum? ....

5. How many cups of milk products are recommended daily? ....

6. What percentage of your daily diet should come from fat? ....

7. What are the most healthy fats?

   ....

8. What types of fat should you avoid or limit?

   ....

   ....

9. What is critical to maintaining a healthy body weight?

   ....

   ....

   ....

10. What is the key to ensuring that your body receives all of the nutrients it needs?

    ....

    ....

    ....

Answers to the Nutrition Quiz

1. Two cups of fruit a day are recommended for a 2,000-calorie diet. Adjust your intake higher or lower depending on your daily calorie level.

2. Two and a half cups of vegetables per day are recommended for a 2,000-calorie diet.

3. The five vegetable subgroups include dark green, orange, legumes, starchy vegetables, and other vegetables. Try to select from each of the five subgroups several times a week.

4. Eat three or more ounce-equivalents of whole-grain products per day.

5. Eat three cups per day of fat-free or low-fat milk or equivalent foods that supply adequate daily dietary calcium.

6. Try to keep total fat consumption to between 20 to 35 percent of total calories. Emphasize healthy fats from sources like fish, nuts, and vegetable oils.

7. Health-enhancing fats come primarily from vegetable oils such as canola, olive, safflower, soybean, and sunflower oils. Fish oils from fatty fish such as salmon and mackerel are also rich in healthy fats.

8. Avoid or limit excess consumption of saturated fats and trans fat. The harder the margarine or shortening, the more likely it is to contain more trans fat. Coconut, palm, and palm kernel oils contain more saturated fat than unsaturated fat.

9. Eat a balanced diet that contains a variety of minimally processed, whole foods and beverages that are rich in nutrients, but low in calories, and balance the amount of food eaten with the amount of activity and energy expended.

10. Eat a variety of foods from all the basic food groups. Limit consumption of saturated and trans fats and added sugars. Avoid processed and highly refined foods. Choose minimally processed, nutrient dense, whole foods in a variety of colors.

Source: Based on The Dietary Guidelines for Americans 2005. Read the full document at www .healthierus.gov/dietary guidelines.

Researchers are currently developing standards for identifying which foods provide the highest nutritional value with the lowest calories. Colorful fruits and vegetables, nuts and beans, whole grains, seafood, low or nonfat dairy foods, and lean meats are more nutrient dense than junk foods such as soft drinks and processed foods that are high calorie and nutrient poor. Among vegetables, spinach and broccoli are more nutrient dense than iceberg lettuce.

Rest and Relax for Best Results

An important, but often overlooked, component of every training program is rest and relaxation. Getting married, however joyful, is a stressful life event. Now, more than ever, it is important that you take time for yourself to rest and to relax. Make it a priority to get a sufficient amount of sleep. Experts recommend that people enjoy anywhere from seven to ten hours per night, depending on individual needs. In addition to sleeping, take time for relaxation. Keep in mind that regardless of how much you want to get in shape for your wedding, it's critical for your health and well-being to not overdo any training program.

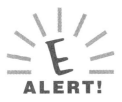
ALERT!

If you're a stressed bride-to-be, exercise is just what you need. There's nothing like a good workout to help you relax and sleep better. Start a solid exercise plan now, and not only will you look your best on your wedding day, you'll be able to blow off steam when you're overloaded from wedding-planning stress.

When you sleep, your body secretes human growth hormone which helps maintain lean muscle mass. Your body also uses this time to repair any cellular damage from training to become stronger. If you skimp on adequate sleep, you're literally accelerating the aging process of your body and preventing yourself from realizing the benefits of your hard work at training.

Relaxation is also very restorative and facilitates healthy weight loss. When you are under stress, your body secretes cortisol into your bloodstream to stimulate your body into a fight or flight state. Studies show that high levels of cortisol contribute to the accumulation of body fat, particularly around the abdominal area, as a protective response for the body. In order to lose weight effectively, you need to reduce feelings of stress and anxiety, which will in turn reduce blood levels of cortisol. Your exercise program can be a great way to alleviate daily stresses. In addition, including mind-body exercises such as yoga, Pilates, and mindful stretching can further help you to restore feelings of calm and inner peace.

Start Celebrating You and Your Love

Your wedding is symbolic of starting a new phase in your life. Making a commitment to putting your best self forward is a wonderful way to mark this occasion. Now that you realize that getting in your best shape is about more than simply tightening your abs, you can take a healthy approach that will provide you and your spouse with dividends for the rest of your lives. The information in this book can support you in your journey of creating your health and happiness, of cherishing the beauty of everyday life, and of looking and feeling your best on your special day.

It is important as you move forward with your exercise program to remember that a healthy body image is essential to a good training program. Individual beauty is in the eye of the beholder, not in digitally enhanced fashion ads. When you incorporate the principles of healthy living, you will achieve your personal best.

Chapter 2
You've Set the Date

Getting ready for your wedding requires much scheduling and organization. You're working with a fixed timeline. You have specific tasks that you must complete. With all of these burdens on your shoulders, the best way to approach your shape-up program is to treat it as valuable time for yourself. In other words, use your training as a much needed time out to take care of you. Your workout time can best be put to use to help relieve stress from extra demands, not as another pressurized item on your to-do list.

Your Training Countdown

Getting visible results from training takes time. While internal changes begin immediately from your very first session, it takes about six to eight weeks for you to see those results in the mirror. You may start to feel better more quickly and notice that you have more energy, sleep better, and are in a better mood, but other adaptations to training require a longer time investment. This is where your commitment to the process of integrating more activity into your lifestyle becomes extremely important.

How to Choose Your Workout Program

Your initial fitness level and how much time you have before your wedding date determine your training approach. This is assuming that you have no medical conditions that require clearance from your health care provider before you get started. The basic workouts in this book are designed for those who are new or returning to fitness after a long period of being inactive. If you haven't been training consistently, it's best to stick with a basic program for at least two months before progressing to intermediate workouts. Otherwise, you risk injuring yourself, which is something you definitely want to avoid before your wedding.

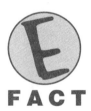

FACT

After consistently training aerobically for four weeks, your body begins to become a more efficient fat burner. Your breathing should become a bit easier during your cardio-workouts and you should notice that you're not huffing and puffing as much when you climb stairs.

The intermediate workouts build upon the base of fitness developed during the initial program. If you're already fit and eager to get started with a more challenging routine, then begin with the intermediate workouts. In the last eight weeks before the important event, move to fine-tuning workouts. Fine-tuning is fun because you focus on the particular assets that you want to emphasize while you wear your wedding dress. For example, you can focus on developing more tone and definition in your shoulders and arms if you're wearing a sleeveless gown.

Before you get started, it's helpful to understand the body's process of physically adapting to the demands of training. With this knowledge, you can anticipate the changes that you will be experiencing. Keep in mind that everyone's response to exercise is individual. Therefore, you may experience these changes at a slightly different rate, depending on your base level of fitness, your age, your physique, whether or not you've been fit in the past, and how often and how hard you train.

Adaptations to Cardio-Training

When you train the cardio-respiratory system, you improve your heart's health and reduce your total amount of body fat. With consistent training over time the heart increases in size. This is positive because a larger heart pumps an increased amount of blood from the heart with every contraction of the heart muscle, resulting in a slower heart beat when you are at rest and a lower blood pressure. These changes can start happening in as few as two weeks or as many as ten weeks of regular training.

Other important physiological changes include the fact that your body becomes more efficient at burning stored fat for fuel and you're able to keep going for longer periods of time. These are key training developments if you want to lose extra weight or to avoid gaining weight over the years. Cardio or aerobic training is important to making your body an efficient burner of fat. Extra fat on your body is nothing more than stored energy. Think of it as extra fuel. In order to use up this extra fuel, you need an efficiently running engine and you need to be able to move for longer periods of time at higher levels of work that uss up more fuel. All of these fuel management changes occur as a direct result of your training.

The primary source of fuel for the body during aerobic exercise is fat. Moderate aerobic exercise, such as a brisk walk for thirty minutes daily, is recommended to maintain health. This walk is also beneficial if it is broken up into three ten minute walks, rather than thirty minutes at a time. If weight loss is a goal, daily walking up to one hour or longer on a cumulative basis is recommended.

Adaptations to Weight Training

When you train your musculoskeletal system, you improve the strength and the endurance of your muscles, you improve your bone density, and you increase your resting metabolic rate, which is the amount of energy or calories that your body burns even when you're sleeping. With consistent training over time, you improve your neuromuscular connection. What that means is that more nerve fibers are connected to your muscles and you can increase the amount of your lean body or muscle mass. These are positive changes. When your neuromuscular system is highly developed, you have more control over your body, and you have more body awareness. When your muscles are stronger and have more endurance, you're able to complete physical tasks with more energy and less fatigue. You reduce your chances of injury and, with stronger bones, you're less likely to experience debilitating and painful bone fractures. You can also avoid the onset of osteoporosis.

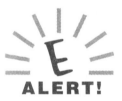

ALERT!

Before fine-tuning your exercise plan, think first things first. You'd never be able to choose the colors of your table linens until you have a reception location, right? So don't zero in on rock-solid abs until you kick into a strong cardio routine. Put the basics in place, then step up to specifics when you're ready.

Muscle conditioning also affects your appearance. More muscle tone gives your body shape and definition. Your physique has more lift rather than droop. Your skin is healthier and has better tone because it receives more circulation from healthy muscles beneath the skin. You look energized and radiant, like a picture of good health.

When you weight train, in contrast to aerobic training, your muscles primarily burn sugar for fuel, also referred to as muscle glycogen. This is positive because you're burning energy. Regardless of whether your body uses fats or uses sugars for fuel, the result at the end of the day is a net deficit if you burn up more energy than you take in. Excess sugars in your body that you don't use for energy are simply converted into stored fat.

Calorie for calorie, the activity of weight training burns as much, if not more, than aerobic training. The difference, however, is we cannot sustain weight training at a continuous level in the way that we can with aerobic training. For example, let's say you can walk consistently without resting for ten, twenty, or thirty minutes. In contrast, you would be absolutely unable to lift any weight for typically more than one minute, at the most two minutes, without the need to take some time out for rest.

With respect to reducing your total amount of body fat, the benefits of weight training for weight management come primarily from two important changes. One, increasing your muscle mass and reducing your overall body fat leads to a higher metabolism (the number of calories that you burn to stay alive). Two, weight training tends to lead to an increase in overall activity levels because you have more energy from your improved muscular strength and endurance. More activity results in more burned calories.

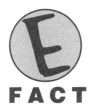

FACT

Studies show the most effective training programs to target weight loss combine both aerobic exercise and strength training. Researchers have compared those who only did only cardio-training, did only weight training, or who combined both for the same time period. Those who did both not only lost the most amount of fat, they also gained the greatest amount of muscle.

Muscle is metabolically more active than fat. It requires a lot more circulation. It is also denser and heavier than fat. Five pounds of muscle is much smaller than five pounds of fat. Therefore, as you begin training, do not be overly concerned with numbers on your scale. It's common for people who begin exercising to actually get smaller in size and stay the same weight or even gain a few pounds. This is a healthy and positive weight gain as it means that you're building more lean body mass. Therefore, do not be too worried about your total weight on the scale. What is more important is your percentage of lean body mass compared to your fat mass.

To see a visible change in muscle tone and definition from weight training requires consistent training, two to three times a week for six to eight weeks. This is because improvements in the mind-body connection through the neuromuscular system must occur first before you see changes in muscle tone or size. Concentrate on the muscles that you're working during each training session to improve results.

At a minimum, therefore, to see visible results from your training, you need to start at least six weeks before your wedding. The more time that you have the better. And, if you start three months, six months, or even one year in advance, you're going to need to pay particular attention in the last six weeks before the big event. For best results, you can use the last six to eight weeks to work on maintaining the fitness level that you have achieved and focus on fine-tuning, rather than general conditioning.

Time and Money: What's It Going to Take?

You'll be happy to know that getting into shape for your wedding doesn't need to be costly or extremely time consuming. As with many things in life, you can choose to spend what you can afford. If you have an unlimited budget, then you can hire a personal trainer, join a gym, or outfit a premium home gym. That would be at the high end. At the lower end of the spectrum, you can buy good workout shoes, a few pieces of equipment, and carve out a space at home to exercise. It's a good idea to set up a space at home that you can use for training even if you also belong to a health club. The reason: you're extremely busy and sometimes, regardless of how hard you try, you won't make it to the gym. The easier it is for you to do your exercise, the more likely it is that you will do it.

In addition to exercise equipment, you need a few essentials regardless of where you exercise. Here, we discuss workout apparel, essentials for outdoor training, and accessories that enhance your training program. For more details about how to set up your home gym, see Chapter 6.

Workout Wear

When it comes to exercise, the right outfit is more than a fashion issue. Today's fitness apparel takes advantage of modern technology to enhance your training comfort and improve performance. For your purposes, comfort and durability should be your priorities when it comes to choosing the right workout wear.

At a minimum, you will require the following:

- One to two pairs of workout shoes
- Several workout tops and bottoms
- Several pairs of cushioned athletic socks
- Three or more exercise bras
- Warm ups or sweats depending on the climate where you live

Your most important investment is your athletic shoes. Good shoes prevent aches and injuries. Go to a specialty sporting goods store for your first purchase to make sure that you get the right fit and style of shoe. Ideally, buy two pairs of shoes so that you can alternate what you wear each day. Because feet sweat during a workout, it's good to allow forty-eight hours for your shoes to become completely dry. This prolongs the life of your shoe and enhances your comfort.

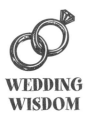

WEDDING WISDOM

You can learn a lot about hunting for a wedding dress from your shoe-shopping excursion. You need to make sure your sneakers are comfortable, and the same goes for your dress. Don't just *walk* around in the dresses you try—sit, stand, turn, and make sure you can breathe! Who knew sequins and sneakers had so much in common?

Keep in mind that your shoes should feel comfortable from the first moment you wear them. You don't need to break in today's shoes. They should feel good and fit well right away. A few things to keep in mind when you go shoe shopping are as follows:

- Bring an old pair of shoes with you, so the salesperson can look at their soles and see what type of shoe you need.
- Go shoe shopping at the end of the day when your feet are at their largest.
- Wear or bring exercise socks.
- Walk around, hop, and jump in the shoes when you try them.

- The shoes should provide cushioning for shock absorption and bend fully at the ball of the foot.
- Ask the salesperson whether you can return them if you wear them once and they hurt your feet. A reputable store will accept such returns.

Buy the style of shoe for the activities that you will be doing. If you plan to wear the same shoes for walking and weight training, you might want to purchase a cross-trainer. Alternatively, if you're a runner and a walker, you might want to purchase a running shoe and a walking shoe that you can also use for your weight training. Discuss these issues with your salesperson. If you have specific foot issues, ask your podiatrist for shoe recommendations.

For information on foot conditions and how to select the right shoe for your feet, go to the American Podiatric Medical Association Web site (*www .apma.org*). The site provides detailed information on foot health and care and even on how to find a podiatrist in your area. Remember, taking care of your feet is essential to an active lifestyle.

Your second most important investment is your sports bra. This is crucial to prevent sagging and to ensure comfort when training. Because most bridal gowns showcase the décolletage, you want to be sure to take good care of yours. Regardless of whether you are an A cup or a triple D or beyond, bras exist to support you. Studies show that the best style for maximal support is an over the shoulder strap bra with separate cup coverage. These provide much better support than the shelf bra designs without cups. If you're particularly busty, you can wear a shelf styled bra over a bra with separate cup coverage. See Appendix D for information on manufacturers of good sports bras.

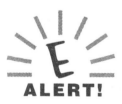

ALERT!

You wouldn't choose any old sports bra to workout, so you can't expect just anything to fit properly under your wedding dress either. Don't wait until the last minute—try several styles under your wedding dress during fittings to make sure your bra does the job right and does not show!

Thirdly, pay attention to technical fabrics. Today's manufacturers have developed fabrics that wick moisture away from the skin and that provide comfortable levels of support. Avoid clothes that are too baggy because they can cause chafing and discomfort.

Outdoor Training Essentials

If you plan to do some of your training outdoors, you not only need to pay attention to your exercise, but you also need to protect yourself from the environment. The number one concern is harmful UVA and UVB rays from the sun. Taking care of your skin with sunscreen is not only good for your health, but it is also an effective strategy to slow down the signs of aging. Remember to cover not only your face, but also your décolletage, shoulders, and arms. Good skincare is essential for a beautiful presentation at your wedding.

You will need the following items for training outdoors:

- Hat or visor with a long and wide brim for sun protection
- Sunglasses
- Broad spectrum sunscreen that protects against UVA and UVB radiation with an SPF 15 or higher
- Reflective vest for walking at dusk, dawn, or in the dark

Clothing can provide some sun protection. Most cotton shirts provide an SPF of about 4 or 6, so you still need to supplement this with sunscreen. In addition to sun protection, you must also make sure that you are visible outdoors to cars and others when you train.

Fun and Valuable Training Accessories

If you have extra funds, treat yourself to training accessories that help keep you motivated, measure your success, and simply make your workouts more fun. The following are supplemental accessories to add to your wish list:

- A digital pedometer that records the number of steps you take daily.
- A scale that measures weight, body composition, and dehydration levels.

- A heart rate monitor to monitor intensity of your cardio-training.
- Some form of portable music player for long walks or runs.

You may even drop a few hints to your friends and family that you'd love any gifts to support your wedding shape-up goals.

Staying Motivated

Getting in shape for your wedding, honeymoon, and new life with your spouse has got to be one of the most motivating goals. At the same time, like any goal, you must achieve it one day and one rep at a time. To keep yourself motivated, you can use some tried and true tips. Research tells that within the first eight weeks of a training program, about 50 percent of people drop out. The usual reason given is lack of time. But one behavioral scientist studied prison inmates who had plenty of time on their hands. As it turned out, in the prison study, about 50 percent of the participant's dropped out. So, what can we conclude from these studies? It's hard to change our habits.

Visualize Your Perfect Day

To keep your motivation high, you need to remind yourself why achieving your goal of being healthy and fit on your wedding day is important to you. Studies show that we're much more likely to make positive choices and change our bad habits if we're fully aware of the benefits that we will receive as a result of sticking with our programs. Take a moment to consider the benefits that you will gain.

Ask yourself the following questions:

- Why do I want to exercise, eat properly, and live healthfully?
- How will my life be better if I become more fit?
- What will be different about how I will feel and look when I'm fit?
- What will be different about the types of things that I will do when I'm fit?
- How will I look and feel on my wedding day when I've achieved my shape-up goals?

Try keeping a journal or writing a letter to yourself. Spell out exactly how you imagine your life will be better as a result of you sticking with your program. When we can really recognize *why* we want to make the tough choices each day to be more active and to eat healthy foods, it's much easier to make the right decisions.

Visualizing your goals makes it easier to achieve them. Post the benefits that you will receive by sticking with your program on your refrigerator or on a bulletin board to serve as a constant reminder. Include pictures of your wedding dress and honeymoon destination to make it even more real for you.

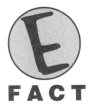

FACT

Planning your wedding and planning to shape up are two things that call for a good dose of realism. Just as you can't expect to coordinate a reception for 200 people in only a few weeks, neither should you expect a complete shape-up so quickly. Give yourself plenty of time to accomplish your goals.

At the same time that you keep the benefits of achieving your goals at the front of your mind, it's also helpful to remember what the negative consequences will be of not making any positive changes. This can also be motivating as a reminder to keep up the good work. Recall that it's hard to make changes in our habits. When the food is delicious, that second portion may be calling you. Those are the moments when you need to remind yourself of why you're going to stop eating when you're full, or that you're still going to take a walk outside even though it's cold.

Getting By with Help from Your Friends

One of the most essential factors to stick successfully with a new exercise, eating, or stress management program is having the support of family and friends. In one study of new exercisers, couples who trained together had a 92 percent success rate of keeping up with their programs. People who trained on their own only had a 55 percent success rate at sticking with their new programs—the typical drop out rate. Recruiting support from the people around you can make all the difference between success and falling by the wayside. Chapter 3 provides lots of tips on training with friends and family, even working out with your dog or a neighbor's dog.

Goal Setting for Success: Short- and Long-Term

You can use a system for setting goals to increase your likelihood of success. Studies show that the best way to achieve a goal is to break it down into small, specific steps that are realistic and achievable. In this manner, you can change your habits gradually. This system is called SMART goal-making.

SMART goals include the following types of goals:

- **Specific:** Perhaps you're having a hard time getting in some aerobic exercise daily. A specific goal would be to walk twenty minutes or more a day.
- **Measurable:** A measurable goal is one that you can evaluate to see whether or not you accomplished it. To make your goal of walking measurable, specify that your goal is to walk a minimum of twenty minutes a day, four days a week. You can objectively verify whether you met this goal.
- **Achievable:** If you haven't been doing any exercise, you don't want to begin with a goal of walking for one hour a day. Start with a goal that you know you can do and focus simply on getting it done.
- **Reasonable:** Achievable and reasonable are closely related concepts. In theory, you may be able to do something, but given the circumstances of your daily life, you cannot do it. For example, if you work eight hours a day, it's not reasonable to assume that you can train three hours a day. Start out by trying to fit in twenty to thirty minutes and build from there.
- **Timed:** Set your goal in a particular time frame. For example, set your goal to walk twenty minutes or more a day, four days a week

for one month. Be sure the time frame you select is specific and that you can verify in your calendar that you did it.

Studies show that SMART goals work. This type of goal-setting allows you to focus on your behaviors and on what you're going to do on a regular basis. It's like the traditional Chinese saying: "The journey of 10,000 miles begins with a single step." To reach your ultimate destination, you need to break down the journey into smaller steps. Travel down your road to success by continuously putting one foot in front of the other.

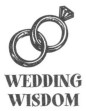

WEDDING WISDOM

With so many details to stay on top of, wedding planning can be overwhelming. When the big picture starts looking too big, adapt the SMART workout plan to suit your wedding routine. Break your plans down into small, specific steps you can tackle in a reasonable time frame, and you'll be more likely to feel you have everything under control.

Try to eliminate threats to your goals before they occur. For example, if environmental cues tend to sabotage you, eliminate them from your surroundings; if you see a bag of cookies and have to eat them all, don't keep bags of cookies in your cupboard. Instead, stock your refrigerator with fresh, sliced fruit or veggies for easy to grab, healthy snacks. Make it easier on yourself.

Rewarding Yourself

Acknowledging your accomplishments and rewarding yourself is also a great way to keep on track. As you look forward to your wedding, you're working hard. Much of your gratification for all of your efforts will not be realized until that important day. Keep your spirits up during the planning period by treating yourself with small rewards each time that you achieve one of your SMART goals.

For example. if you were able to walk five times a week for twenty minutes or more for two weeks, plan on treating yourself to something that you enjoy. It can be something to pamper yourself, such as a massage, pedicure, or manicure. Or, you can choose a recreational activity that you enjoy—tickets to a show that you've been wanting to see. It doesn't need to be expensive. Your reward should represent something special that you do for yourself that is not part of your daily life—a simple way to give yourself a well-deserved pat on the back.

Overcoming Bumps in the Road

In addition to planning mini-steps along the way to achieving your grander goals, you need to plan for those times that you can't or won't be able to stick to your plans. In other words, instead of being unrealistic and thinking that every week is going to flow smooth as clockwork, create backup plans for those times when you won't be able to go to the gym or to take a walk around the block. Bumps in the road of life are normal. If you have some backup plans, you're much more likely to be successful in the long-term, than if you expect that you'll always be able to stick to your routine.

People who are most successful at achieving goals do not let mistakes prevent them from trying again. Instead of beating yourself up or giving up on your program, learn from why a particular plan of action or mini-goal did not work for you. Those who ultimately succeed are those who learn from mistakes and try again to be successful.

Chapter 3

Keys to Training Success

Learning how to integrate activity and exercise into daily living is essential, because if you can't overcome that hurdle, you won't find time to workout. One of the keys to training success is to realize that your exercise program is only one part of your overall goal of bringing more wellness into your being. People are often derailed when they become stressed. They throw out their workouts, give up on good nutrition, and fall back on bad habits. Staying focused on wellness helps you to stay motivated and on track.

Aiming for Wellness and Self-Care

Living well is as much about your attitude as it is about the choices that you make. You create your health and well-being each and every day with small decisions such as eating fresh fruits and vegetables, moving your body more, treating others and yourself with kindness, and honoring and respecting the needs of your body to rest, relax, and exercise. Success in cultivating a healthy lifestyle depends a great deal on your attitude, your self-esteem, your skill at juggling priorities, and your capacity for finding joy and pleasure in the present.

Your Positive Attitude

A strong and healthy mind contributes to a strong and healthy body. More and more studies show that the power of positive thinking is genuine. People who believe that they're able to accomplish a goal are much more likely to succeed in achieving it. Some studies show that people with more positive attitudes even have stronger immune systems, are more able to fight off infections successfully, and are less likely to come down with illnesses.

With your impending marriage and change in your life's circumstances, you're facing a time when multiple demands are being placed upon you. The decisions that you make not only affect you, but also your future family, closest friends, and future spouse. To overcome these pressures and handle your responsibilities well, it's important to remind yourself that you're doing the best that you can and that you're only human. In other words, don't put superhuman demands or expectations upon yourself. Be sure to take extra time for pampering and self-care.

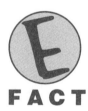

FACT

Relaxation is essential to your well-being and also to successful weight management. When you're stressed, you secrete the hormone cortisol. This hormone contributes to the accumulation of fat, particularly in the abdominal area. To reduce weight in this area, you need to lower your levels of stress hormones as well as exercise and eat right.

Instead of focusing on what you can't do and thereby increasing your stress levels, stay positive about what you're able to fit into your schedule. Everything and anything that you do is a step in the right direction. If you can't do a forty-five minute workout, don't beat yourself up. Negative, self-defeating thoughts do much more harm than good. Turn the situation around and do a fifteen-minute workout and be glad that you could squeeze that much in. Each day, try to find time for a few minutes of something good for your body—deep breathing, stretching, walking, a set of pushups or squats—whatever you can integrate into your daily routine.

When you're not able to be as active as you like, stay on course with your wellness goals and eat plenty of healthy foods that day. Add more salads and fresh fruit to your plate in place of things that are high in fat or sugar or that are highly processed. Give yourself time for relaxing activities, such as enjoying a bubble bath by candlelight. Or, go to bed early and catch up on your sleep. All of these actions help you to achieve your fitness and wellness goals, because you'll wake up refreshed and motivated the next morning. In this manner, you can find success each and every day.

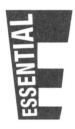

Achieving success is the single most important factor to building self-confidence, which helps ensure more accomplishments. You need to set realistic goals for yourself to reinforce your ability to be successful. Positive role models help you to believe in your ability to do well. Seek out the company of friends who follow the lifestyle that you want to create for yourself.

Pay attention to how you talk to yourself. Negative self-talk can undermine your best efforts. Notice if you criticize or judge yourself, or engage in "all or nothing" thinking. An example of this is, "I missed my workout today so I might as well eat a pint of ice cream." This type of mindset tends to escalate feelings of guilt and undermines your resolve to get back on track. Use the strategies described above to keep yourself positive about your ability to take good care of yourself each and every day. Congratulate and celebrate all the great things that you do *right*. Forgive yourself when you're not perfect. Learn from the situation and simply let it go.

Do What Works for You

This book is packed with ideas, exercises, programs, and tips on how to shape up for your wedding day. But remember, you don't have to do or use every single one of them! Pick and choose among all the suggestions and go with what works for you. Make an effort to individualize your program. In other words, when what you decide to do meshes easily with what you want to achieve and with how you enjoy spending your time, then you're much more likely to meet with success. So, take the time to figure out what is actually achievable for you and what you like to do.

Your body has an inner wisdom. Cultivate your ability to hear your own internal messages more strongly. Pay attention to what feels good and right for your body and what feels uncomfortable or awkward. Notice whether you feel refreshed and energized after you complete an exercise sequence. If it helps you, track your feelings in a journal. After you've accumulated some entries, read what you've written and see if you can detect any patterns in your activities, your energy levels, and your feelings of well-being.

Another important step for you is to take full responsibility for your program. All of this information is here to support you. Ultimately, however, no one can execute any of these actions except you. No one but you can create your own health.

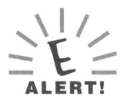

ALERT!

Studies show that it takes a minimum of two months to develop a new habit. If you find it challenging to keep up with your workout goals those first eight weeks, hang in there. Use as many strategies as possible to create a routine of more activity for yourself. After those first two months, you'll find it much easier to maintain.`

The bottom line: stay focused on what really matters. You're getting married. You want all of your wedding festivities to commemorate this momentous occasion. You want to celebrate your love and share this experience with those who are nearest and dearest to you. With that in mind, keep your training in perspective. Be realistic about what you can achieve with the amount of time that you have available. Do your best and be proud of yourself.

Enjoy the Process

Your wedding workout program is not simply about end results and achieving goals; it's about enjoying the process. It's about feeling pleasure and joy in movement as an affirmation of your own sense of aliveness. It's about releasing your stress and tension and enjoying a deep and good night's sleep. It's about living life fully and being the best person that you can, because it makes you feel good about who you are. You're taking important steps toward your own self-care, which will also help your spouse and your future life together. Your best self lies within you. You're actively taking steps to highlight that part of yourself.

Enjoy your training program as part of the whole series of events that will culminate with your wedding. And, the best part is that you can continue maintaining your fitness and enjoying wellness in your life long after the wedding and honeymoon are over.

Positive Body Image

To get the best results from any training program, you need to begin by loving and appreciating yourself and your body. Many of us look in the mirror and judge ourselves. We feel disappointed that we don't look like models in magazines or celebrities on television. We're frustrated with the way a natural body looks. Our society puts a premium value on physical perfection, so it's no wonder we feel discouraged when our bodies don't match up to that ideal. Healthy bodies come in many different shapes and sizes. Your body is a marvelous miracle. It allows you to do the work you are meant to do, care for those you love, and feel great sensual pleasure. Your body makes the experience of your life possible. Respecting your body means appreciating all that it has done and continues to do for you. Love and accept it. Be patient. Only when you feel self-acceptance can you make true gains in strength—not only physical strength but also inner strength from your own sense of purpose and value.

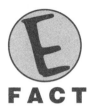

FACT

Wedding planning is a huge endeavor—not only is getting married one of the most momentous events in your life, your reception is probably the biggest celebration you've ever had to plan. Coordinating all of the little details is bound to get stressful at times. Finding positive outlets like exercise to help you cope with your stress is a must.

Respecting your body also means that you take the necessary time to learn basic exercises and build a conditioning base before you progress to a more difficult program. Take one level at a time, gradually train the correct muscles, focus your mind, body, and spirit, and you'll eventually be able to do more advanced programs. This process requires discipline, but the benefits are worth it. The wonderful thing about the human body is that if you practice consistently, you will become stronger. So, take your time, and have faith in the process.

Overcoming Training Myths and Misconceptions

Equally important as a positive attitude is the need to clear up the many misconceptions and myths that surround the exercise and training process. We're bombarded by advertisements that guarantee "amazing" results from gadgets in only minutes a day or pills that "melt" fat off our bodies. If it were truly that simple, wouldn't everyone be fit? Clearly, quick fixes are not the answer.

This misinformation does a serious disservice to people. Achieving health, fitness, and wellness is not complex, but it isn't something that is acquired instantly. It requires a lifestyle of healthy living that includes sensible amounts of activity, eating healthy foods in moderate portions, getting enough sleep to feel rested and restored, spending time with family and friends, and relaxing and enjoying pursuits that are meaningful and fulfilling.

The following are common misconceptions about exercise:

- **No pain, no gain:** *Moderate* exercise prevents injury and produces results.
- **Exercise is only for athletes:** The human body is designed to move. Modern living requires us to exercise because most natural activity is no longer necessary. Every person benefits from exercise and moderate levels of daily activity.
- **Weight training makes you big:** Very few people have the genetics necessary to build large muscles naturally and certain styles of training build more muscle size than others. Moderate levels of weight training improve your muscle conditioning and are good for your bones and joints.
- **Weight training doesn't help you lose weight:** The most successful programs for weight loss and maintenance include a combination of weight training, aerobic exercise, and good nutrition.
- **One type of exercise is better than others:** Exercise enthusiasts swear by yoga or weight training, or whatever it is that they love to do. The best training program includes a combination of activities.
- **If you exercise a lot, it doesn't matter what you eat:** While it's true that if you're very active you can eat more food without gaining weight because you're using lots of energy, the best diet still consists primarily of fruits, vegetables, whole grains, and other fresh and minimally processed foods.
- **You shouldn't exercise when you have your period:** Female Olympians have won gold medals when they have their periods. How you feel is your best judge. You should avoid anything inverted, such as a headstand. Light exercise helps many women to feel better.
- **Taking a supplement can make you slim and fit:** No supplement exists that can replace the benefits of a balanced exercise program and good nutrition. The bottom line: save your money.

Getting to the bottom of these false notions can help you to realize your true dreams. Once you clear up these false beliefs, you can take solid steps toward real solutions to achieving what you want to create in your life.

Increasing Your Lifestyle Activity

An underestimated but extremely powerful way to improve your health, burn more energy, and effectively manage your weight is to increase your daily activity. That means if you move more each and every day, it can do more for you than going to the gym two or three times a week. According to a 1999 study, increasing lifestyle physical activity is equally as effective as a structured exercise program in improving exercise, cardio-respiratory fitness, and blood pressure.

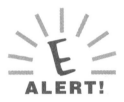

ALERT!

Research shows that people who have a lot of excess weight tend to sit more than their thinner counterparts. One study found that "naturally" leaner individuals moved more, while heavier people sat 150 minutes more per day and consequently burned 350 less calories per day. Simply getting up out of the chair and moving more can make a big difference.

You can benefit from these study findings by brainstorming more ways that you can be active in your day-to-day routine. Especially as your wedding date grows nearer, you'll have less and less time for structured exercise activities. You can compensate for that by fitting in more daily movement.

Here are some suggestions to help you move more day after day:

- Park farther away from your office, shops, and your own front door.
- Get off one station earlier from the train or bus and walk the remainder.
- Take the stairs instead of the elevator. In multiple story buildings, take the elevator to one or two floors below your destination and walk the rest.
- Avoid moving sidewalks; walk on the regular floor instead.
- When you go grocery shopping, walk down all of the aisles.
- Return shopping carts back to the store.

- When you go to the shopping mall, do an extra lap around the main strip.
- Meet friends for walking dates instead of for coffee.
- Try walking meetings with colleagues instead of sitting in the office.
- Stand and pace when you're on the telephone.
- Deliver a message in person instead of sending an e-mail.
- Send your documents to a printer that is on the other side of the office.
- Find an office colleague to walk with at lunchtime a few days a week, or walk alone.
- Take multiple trips when you clear the table or do other household chores.
- Do a set of pushups at the sink after you brush your teeth.
- Do a set of squats before you sit in your chair in front of the computer.
- Take stairs two at a time for a set of lunges.

These are a few ideas to give you some food for thought. Take some time with your journal or with your friends to brainstorm more ways that you can add activity into your day. The average-sized woman burns approximately one calorie per minute when sitting. Simply by standing upright, she doubles her energy expenditure. Marching in place burns three calories per minute, and slow pacing equals four calories per minute. Find every opportunity to stand instead of sit, march instead of stand, and pace instead of march. Every step adds up to make a powerful difference. Wear a pedometer to record your daily movements and aim for up to 10,000 to 15,000 steps daily.

Training with the Groom and Bridal Attendants

Having the support of your friends, family, and your fiancé to help you achieve your wellness goals is a very effective strategy for success. It's difficult to make changes in isolation. If you recruit the support of those around you by letting them know how important it is to you to improve your nutritional and exercise habits, they can make a huge difference.

Numerous studies show that the single most important ingredient for success with sticking to a new exercise and eating regimen is the support of friends and family.

Don't be shy about what you want to accomplish. Announce the fact that you're working out and improving your health habits to all your friends. Let them know that you'd love their help and support. You'll be amazed at the difference that it will make. Your friends can reinforce your accomplishments, encourage you to stay on track, compliment you on your discipline, and tell you things that you need to hear to keep you motivated.

Recruit your friends and family as training buddies. Some of your bridal attendants may share your goals of wanting to get in shape. When you need to catch up or go over wedding details, instead of getting together over food and drinks, get together for a walk or a workout. Find different ways that you can be active together. You can visit studios or exercise classes as a group or even chip in and share a personal trainer. Small group training is growing in popularity. Alternatively, you can meet up for hikes on the weekend or other outdoor nature walks. Explore different ways to spend active quality time jointly.

Invite your fiancé to participate in your wellness goals as well. Do some evening stretches as partners to help both of you relax and unwind at the end of the day. If you're not sure how to do them, read the instructions to each other and practice. You can also take walks together to discuss plans and things that you need to resolve before the wedding.

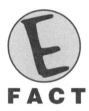

FACT

Studies show that men and women who are more fit tend to have sex more often and experience greater satisfaction with their sex lives. Research also shows that maintaining an active sex life enhances both the quality and length of life.

At the same time, amidst all the stress of wedding organization, don't forget to have fun times with your fiancé. Being active together can be a great way to bond, fit in more exercise, and relieve some of the pressures of all the things you need to get done before the big day. Think of classes that you may be able to take jointly or other ways that you can spend time in each other's company and keep moving.

Make time to play together. Indulge in some things just for fun, without any wedding planning purpose. Spend time in nature, run on the beach or take a hike in the woods. Plan an outing to a park together, go skating, or do anything active—purely for the fun of it and no other reason.

Training with a Dog

Don't forget the pleasure of spending time together with a dog. If you don't own a dog, borrow a neighbor's or a friend's pet for an easy stroll. Dogs relish the chance to burn off extra energy and are happier and more relaxed with regular exercise. Studies show that people who walk dogs regularly are more successful at losing weight and keeping it off than those who simply walk on their own.

Here are some tips for healthy and enjoyable dog walking:

- Make sure the dog has no medical conditions that prevent increasing exercise. Wait a minimum of one hour after meals. Large dogs, in particular, can experience bloating from air filling up their stomachs. Serious cases can cause shock or even death.
- Check terrain for any hazards that can harm dog paws such as broken glass, nails, stakes, wires, metal fragments, holes, or ditches. Walk on soft grass or dirt paths if they're available.
- Keep the dog at your side in the "heel" position or slightly in front of you.
- In warm weather, be alert to any signs of heat exhaustion or heat stroke from your dog, such as heavy panting, hanging tongue, altered gait, or other signs of fatigue.
- On cold days, dogs with short, thin fur can get chilled. Add a doggie sweater if you notice any shivering.
- After walks, check paws and paw pads for cracks, sores, cuts, or any debris between toes, especially if you observe any limping or stiff or pained movements. Keep claws trimmed.

If your dog misbehaves, consider taking an obedience class together. You'll both benefit from learning the proper commands to use during walks. Walking a dog is a great way to take your mind off other issues as you both explore and discover the outdoors together. If you don't own a dog and don't know anyone else who owns one either, check out your local Humane Society or Society for the Prevention of Cruelty to Animals. Many times these organizations have walking programs where you can "borrow" shelter dogs and take them out for a walk, which benefits everyone!

Chapter 4
The Less-Stressed Bride

Stress is very familiar to every bride-to-be. Stress can give you the adrenaline push to get through all the heavy demands on your time during this pre-wedding push. However, if unmanaged, stress can undermine your pleasure, your health, your effectiveness, and your relationships during this critical time period. In this chapter, you will learn what stress is, how stress undermines your health and shape-up efforts, how you can identify stress, and what steps you can take to reduce stress and restore balance to your life.

What Is Stress?

Stress is a natural physiological response to something that triggers a feeling of fear or threat. The purpose of this response, called "fight or flight," is to help us to survive life-threatening situations. The natural chemical reaction that affects your mind and body is like a miracle drug that can save your life in the face of an emergency. For example, if your house catches on fire in the middle of the night, stress can help you to think quickly and effectively the minute you wake up. As soon as you realize you're in danger, stress gives you energy to jump out of bed and run for your life. You have extra strength to save loved ones who may be in danger. In an instant, your mind is alert, your heart is pounding, your muscles are strong, and you have superhuman energy.

The Stress Response

The body's response to stress is stimulated by stress hormones, such as adrenalin and cortisol, which are released by your body to prepare you for action. Among other things, these stress hormones do the following:

- Increase your heart rate and blood pressure to pump an extra burst of oxygen-rich blood through your body so you can get moving
- Constrict arteries to stop the flow of blood to your digestive system and skin
- Relax arteries to increase blood flow to the brain and muscles
- Trigger sugar release into your bloodstream for quick energy
- Increase perspiration to cool the body
- Speed up your breathing rate and open bronchial tubes to draw more oxygen-rich air into the lungs

When you look at all of these changes, it's easy to see how this chemically induced state of emergency preparedness is extremely useful in life-threatening situations.

Today's challenge, however, is to manage the stress response, which may be triggered when you're not in any physical danger at all. In fact, most modern stresses are mental and emotional. You find yourself stuck in traffic, missing deadlines for wedding preparations, getting ready to face all your relatives, or worrying that your friends and family won't get along at the reception. If you're under a lot of pressure juggling your work, your wedding preparations, your friends and family, and your efforts to get ready for your new life together, these stress levels stay high each day. Your body and mind feel the strain, and your body has no opportunity to physically release any of this tense energy.

Unmanaged Stress

Stress can be unhealthy if it mounts to levels at which you feel that you can no longer cope. This usually occurs after stress levels have remained high over a prolonged period of time.

Physical and mental symptoms of excessive stress include:

- High blood pressure
- Rapid pulse
- Chronic muscle tension
- Headaches
- Digestive problems
- Irritability
- Depression
- Anxiety
- Loss of ability to concentrate
- Altered sleeping or eating habits
- Increased use of drugs or alcohol

High stress can even increase the risk of a heart attack. Understanding stress and having skills to manage stress effectively, therefore, is important to your overall health and wellness and will come in particularly handy during this pre-wedding period.

Managing Stress for a Better Shape-Up

Learning how to manage stress is important to your shape-up program because most people fail to achieve their shape up and weight management goals when too much stress disrupts their life. When stress levels mount, people often turn to unhealthy habits to help them cope, such as overeating comfort foods, drinking excessive amounts of alcohol, or smoking. Instead of using exercise as a positive way to manage stress, all thoughts of exercising are forgotten.

In recent studies, researchers have found a relationship to the accumulation of fat in the abdominal area of the body and high stress levels. Scientists theorize that when the body believes that it is in a state of stress, it holds on to fat as a source of protection. Historically, this would have been beneficial if famines, wars, extreme environmental conditions, or food shortages caused the stress. In our modern world, however, most stressful conditions exist in a setting where food is abundant, not scarce.

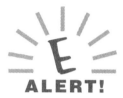

ALERT!

For people with diabetes, stress can negatively affect managing blood glucose levels. While individuals differ, people with Type 2 diabetes find that stress often increases blood glucose. Since high levels of blood glucose can also damage blood vessels, it's particularly important for people with diabetes to effectively manage stress.

While it's counter-intuitive, worrying about losing weight and getting in shape is not productive. In fact, not only is it not productive, it undermines your positive efforts. Instead, what is more helpful is focusing on a positive attitude, learning how to identify and manage stress, and cultivating healthy habits such as exercising when you feel wound up and relaxing when you feel very exhausted and drained.

Identifying Stress in Your Life

Planning your wedding does include meeting many deadlines, negotiating with many different personalities, and juggling numerous relationships successfully. While this does not necessarily have to be stressful, it can be if you feel overwhelmed, particularly if you are also managing a full-time career. If you feel frequently rushed or pressured and feel overwhelmed by this, you let small frustrations get to you, or you find it hard to forget your worries and relax, tackling your stress is likely to improve your health and enhance your success with your shape-up program. At the same time, you can certainly make your life more enjoyable, at least for you and your future spouse.

Other types of stress are not caused by your attitude, but are rather the product of a busy life. For example, if you are driving in heavy traffic and someone quickly cuts in front of you, that might be a stressful situation. You have a legitimate fear for your safety because a car accident could result. Your reaction, however, does not require you to burn off any physical energy. Rather, you remain seated in your car. You're likely to tighten your muscles and experience feelings of tension and anxiety as your body undergoes the physiological and biochemical changes associated with the fight or flight response.

Determining Causes

One of the first steps to learning how to manage stress effectively is to identify the individual pressures—the types of things in your life that cause you stress. The next time you start to feel overwhelmed and stressed out, explore these feelings in greater depth. Ask yourself the following questions to determine what is causing you to feel this way:

- Am I overcommitted?
- Am I taking care of others and neglecting my own self-care?
- Am I trying to accomplish everything on my own without asking for any support from anyone else?
- Are my expectations unrealistic?
- What is going on in my life right now that gives me a sense of struggle?

If you're keeping a journal, try to record things that trigger your stress. You can include these items with the other information that is relevant to your workout progress. Write down the stressful event that happened, what you were thinking or feeling, and how you reacted physically. This can give you valuable insight into the cumulative triggers you face throughout the day.

Identifying Priorities

When people feel stressed out, they often also feel frustrated—as if they're not able to accomplish the things that they feel are important to them. The following is a valuable exercise to help you get in touch with what you want to achieve and how you are actually spending your time. First, write down the top five things that you want to accomplish in your life these days and how they relate to your overall values. For example, one of your top priorities may be to manage all of your wedding preparations to create an unforgettable experience that will memorialize the celebration of your love and your life together with your fiancé. This relates to the value that you place on your personal life and your relationships with friends and family.

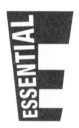

Here's a quick trick to take the edge off during stressful wedding-planning situations: Breathe deeply all the way into your stomach, fill up with air through your diaphragm, then bring the air up through your lungs and into your chest. A few deep "three-part" breaths like these will help you to keep your cool and keep your blood pressure down.

Next, write down how you spend your waking hours during a typical day on a percentage basis. For example, if you sleep eight hours a day, then you have sixteen hours remaining. Each hour represents approximately 6 percent of your day. So, if you spend three hours per day eating, that is 18 percent of your day. And, if you spend two hours per day commuting, that is 12 percent of your day. Work on this breakdown until you can get to an accounting of approximately 100 percent of how you spend your time on a typical day.

Most people discover that they are not spending any time whatsoever on items that they have identified as important to them, such as being active on a regular basis. Many people realize they have not allocated any time at all to self-care. If you want to achieve certain goals in your life, you need to make time for them in your schedule. Doing this exercise helps you to be aware of why you may not be achieving some of the things that you want. Now, you can start the brainstorming process to see how you can be more efficient with your time and how you can strategize so that each day brings you closer to your particular goals such as good health, fitness, and well-being.

Stress Management Tips

It's important for your health and mental wellness that you feel a sense of control over your life. Stress management is a learned skill; successful stress management requires strategic planning. You can make a difference. It simply requires a little concentrated effort. The strategies discussed in this section can help you cope with the stress in your life more effectively.

Effective Time Management

Developing time management skills is critical to successfully manage stress. Everyone has the same number of hours in the day. Some people, however, are more effective managers of their time and priorities. To get organized, first identify your priorities and then identify your time wasters. Maybe you simply don't need to watch as much television as you do, or you can combine your commuting with some other tasks.

Next, make a realistic plan for how long it will take you to get the things that are important to you accomplished. You can use the SMART goal setting process described in Chapter 2. Consider your workout goals in the context of the rest of your life. If you don't have time to go to the gym, don't plan to do it. You'll only set yourself up for disappointment. Instead, spend your time brainstorming how you can add more walking into your normal daily schedule, to the office, on your breaks, and at the end of the day. Fit in some toning and stretching in the morning and in the evening. Do the best that you can, and remember to also leave time for yourself.

Get Help from Friends and Family

Social support is a critical factor in effective stress management. Friends and family can help you to talk over troublesome topics and help you keep your perspective. Take time to spend with your friends and family and to maintain relationships. Even a cherished pet can provide you with companionship and dispel feelings of loneliness and isolation.

If you feel that you need more support, go ahead and ask for help from others in your home, workplace, or community. Don't try to do everything alone. If you ask, you'll realize that many people are there for you and are more than willing to lend assistance.

Don't Sweat the Small Stuff

If you find that you are often irritated or annoyed, this can be a sign that your stress levels are too high. Learn constructive methods to deal with disagreeable situations. Remind yourself that effective communication can often defuse many conflicts. Make sure that you're not allowing resentment to build up inside you. Over time, denial of anger can lead to unhealthy blowups or chronic negative feelings. The healthiest approach is to learn how to effectively express your feelings in positive and constructive ways.

It may help to remember some simple alternatives to becoming angry or frustrated in stressful situations. If possible, leave the scene of a stressful situation before it gets to you. Talk to someone you trust about how you feel, or take some time on your own to brainstorm nonstressful ways to respond to a stressful issue. Most importantly, remember to breathe deeply, and ask yourself, "In the grand scheme of things, does this really matter?"

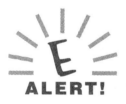

Unchecked stress takes its toll on more than just your emotional state. It eventually manifests as physical symptoms—from muscle strains and spasms, to more serious injuries or illnesses. Your body will let you know when it's under too much stress, so listen!

Get Active Outside

A great way to restore calm and your sense of perspective, as well as to fit in some healthy activity, is to get outside and enjoy nature. Studies show that spending time in nature promotes feelings of calm and relaxation. When you look at a beautiful sunset, listen to the sounds of the pounding surf, or take in a beautiful view from the side of a mountain, it helps to put all the small frustrations back in the proper perspective. Find something active outside that you enjoy, and take time to put it in your schedule.

Keep in mind that your exercise does not always need to take place in a gym and it does not always have to be a formal workout. Sometimes, a quick refreshing walk in a park can be extremely restorative as well as provide you with healthful activity. Not only will you feel better, look great, and manage your weight effectively, but you'll also manage stress better by being active regularly. Something as simple as a short walk can be a powerful positive outlet for tension. Use your active time as a stress reliever and not as another pressurized "to-do" on your already loaded schedule.

Make Time for Self-Care

One of the biggest contributors to feelings of stress is the sense that life is out of control. To avoid this, make time for yourself. You deserve time for your own self-care. For one thing, it supports your health, which in turn helps you to better support all the people you care about. Take a moment to identify things that you enjoy, and that are fun and restorative. Make it a point to incorporate these activities into your schedule.

It's never easy to change a habit. Unless stress is managed and the reasons for maintaining the behavioral change are foremost in your mind, old habits prevail. A calm, clear, and focused mind and a healthy, realistic attitude are important for achieving any goal. This holds true for the incorporation of healthy lifestyle habits too. Don't judge yourself or beat yourself up if you find that you're not always exercising. Simply take a deep breath and get back to doing the things that you know will make you feel better and help you to enjoy life more.

Restoring Balance—Making Time to Relax

Relaxation techniques can be used to counteract the effects of stress on your mind and body, with significant health benefits. Regular relaxation can reduce blood cortisol levels, blood pressure, cholesterol, and blood glucose.

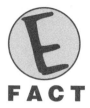

FACT

Studies show that relaxation can reduce headaches, pain, anxiety, and menopausal symptoms. At the same time, it can enhance healing, immune cell response, concentration, and feelings of well-being. Relaxation has even been shown to improve fertility rates in infertile women.

Research done in the 1970s by Dr. Herbert Benson of Harvard University began to explore the relationship between mental techniques and physiological effects. Benson studied people who participated in transcendental meditation. He coined the term *the relaxation response,* which is defined as "a calm state brought about by sitting quietly and repeating a sound, word, or muscular activity over and over. When everyday thoughts intrude, the person passively disregards them and returns to the repetition." The relaxation response reflects a physiological state brought about by reducing stress and calming the mind.

The relaxation response produces the following effects:

- Lower blood pressure
- Slower heart rate
- Slower breathing rate
- Return of blood flow to the skin and extremities
- Less perspiration
- Release of muscular tension

When you look at the results of the relaxation response and compare them to the stress response list at the beginning of this chapter, it's easy to see how relaxation counteracts stress and restores the body to a balanced state.

Make time to explore and learn techniques that help you to relax. Some people use prayer, while others meditate or engage in practices like yoga or tai chi. Find the methods that work best for you.

A good strategy is to combine an active relaxation or stress reducing technique such as walking, dancing, or weight training with a quiet relaxation technique such as deep breathing or meditation. The active technique can help you let go of the pent up energy from the stimulation of the stress response and help you burn off some of the excess tension. The quiet technique can then help you to calm, quiet, and center yourself, and bring you back to your inner sense of peace and balance.

Studies show that people who learn effective stress management techniques are much more successful at achieving long-lasting behavioral change in the areas of increased physical activity, improved nutrition, smoking cessation, and weight management.

Relaxation, Deep Breathing, and Meditation

One of the easiest ways to achieve relaxation is to engage in deep, mindful breathing exercises. This can help trigger the relaxation response. This type of exercise is easy to learn, quick to perform, and requires no equipment. It is also a good introduction to learning how to meditate. As you continue to explore other methods of relaxation, use the following breathing exercise to ease tensions and restore your sense of balance and calm. It will do the health of your body, mind, and spirit a world of good. As you emerge from your restorative relaxation time, remind yourself that you have the power to create your own health and to enjoy all that life has to offer to you.

A Simple Breathing Exercise

This exercise is an excellent introduction to relaxation and to meditation techniques. It increases self and body awareness. A two- to three-minute "breathing break" during the day is very restorative. To perform this simple exercise, sit or lie comfortably with your hands resting in your lap. Relax your muscles and close your eyes.

Make no effort to control your breath. Simply breathe naturally. As you breathe in and out, focus your attention on the breath and how the body moves with each inhalation and exhalation.

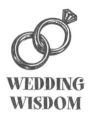

WEDDING WISDOM

Weddings can be stressful because they usher in huge life changes and stir up emotions. You and your groom will be adjusting to newly married life, but don't forget your family and friends—things will change for them, too. Do yourself and those you love a favor: Get to the heart of any issues you're having *before* you walk down the aisle.

Take a few moments to focus inward. Notice the movement of your body as you breathe. Observe your inhalation and exhalation. Pay particular attention to how the breath moves your body. Observe your chest, shoulders, rib cage, and stomach. Notice subtleties such as whether your chest or stomach rises with inhalation and how your body responds to exhalation. Don't try to control your breath, simply focus your attention on it. This singular focus brings you into the present moment and into the immediate experience of your body. It often results in slower, deeper breaths that further relax your body.

If thoughts come into your mind, simply let them come and go. Allow the thoughts to drift by like clouds floating in the sky. Any time your mind begins to wander, return your attention to your breathing. Continue for two to three minutes and then gently open your eyes. Over time, you can lengthen the period of relaxation, if you prefer.

Benefits of Meditation

Doing deep breathing exercises on a regular basis is great preparation for beginning a meditation practice. Millions of Americans practice meditation to improve their sense of well-being and more and more research is substantiating its health benefits. Simply put, meditation is a discipline of training and focusing the mind, similar to the way that fitness is an approach to training and disciplining the body. For example, a person who lacks knowledge of the tools and methods of fitness may think that his or her lack of strength, endurance, or energy are inevitable, rather than aspects of life that can be changed with consistent training and a healthy lifestyle. Similarly, a person with an untrained mind may think that the constant stream of random thoughts, emotions, and unthinking reactions to circumstances are the result of personality, rather than thinking of them as aspects of life that can be changed.

People who adopt a fitness and health lifestyle often experience feelings of empowerment and self-esteem, because they are able to exert greater control over their own bodies. Similarly, people who practice meditation often experience feelings of well-being and calm, because they discover that they possess much greater depth and inner balance above the mindless chatter. In other words, a mentally trained person knows that random thoughts and emotions are always drifting by. Instead of reacting impulsively, a calm and centered person can live with a more open awareness of present experience and can respond to life's pressures with thoughtful choices. In other words, people who meditate regularly have more control over their own minds.

Establishing a Meditation Practice

If you want to develop a meditation practice, begin by practicing deep breathing on a regular basis at a consistent time each day. Begin with a few minutes of practice and work up to longer periods of time. If you don't want to do a seated meditation, you can practice this mindful focus and attention to breathing during a walking meditation. For effective walking meditation, quiet and focus your mind on all the sensations of walking. Again, if your mind wanders, simply bring it back to your breathing and to your experience of walking in the present moment. You'll find that when you finish your meditative walk, you'll feel as refreshed as if you've taken a long, restorative nap.

The presence of stress in our lives gives us an awareness of the depth of our mind and body connection and how our thoughts and feelings affect our physical well-being. In addition, learning how to release this tension and restore feelings of well-being shows us how our body can also affect our mind and our feelings. Science is now substantiating the theory that we have the power within us to manifest both outer *and* inner health. Meditation and other relaxation techniques provide you with an opportunity to create more health, peace, and balance in your life and in the lives of those you love. Your time and efforts dedicated to taking care of the stress in your life will deliver significant rewards.

Chapter 5

Saying "I Do" to Healthy Eating

Your healthy eating habits are a key ingredient to your success in looking picture perfect on your wedding day and beyond. Exercise is important, but if you don't combine it with good nutrition you'll have a harder time seeing results. Your skin, hair, and energy all reflect what you eat. This chapter helps you to achieve a healthier pattern of eating with nutritional tips, menu planning ideas, and recommendations for dining out that all help you avoid sabotaging your best intentions.

Good Nutrition for Your Wedding Shape-Up

A nutritious diet is one of the single most important keys to creating your long-term health and it is the cornerstone of your wedding workout program. The old adage, "You are what you eat," is truly the bottom line. Foods that you consume provide your body with all of its nutrients—the building blocks for your physical repair and growth—and all of its fuel—the energy supply for your activities.

Food, Nutrition, and Appearance

The connection between what you eat and your body's composition (ratio of fat to nonfat weight), appearance, and health is direct. Overeating foods, particularly those that are high in processed sugar and animal fat, leads to excess amounts of stored fuel on your body in the form of fat. When humans lived in nature, stored fat provided a source of protection from famine and ensured survival. In the United States today, however, food is abundant and people move much less. Therefore, we need less fuel to get us through our daily activities and we certainly don't need to carry spare fuel around.

Selecting Foods

To manage your weight and optimize your health effectively, you must keep in mind two important points about the foods that you select. First, seek out nutrient rich foods, those that contain vitamins, minerals, antioxidants, fiber, and other nutrients. Second, choose foods that are low in energy as measured in calories, while still high in nutrition. For example, a processed cookie that is high in sugar and fat (energy) is low in vitamins, minerals, and other essential nutrients. In contrast, organic nuts or olive oil would also be high in fat but also very high in essential nutrients that are particularly beneficial to your health. Similarly, broccoli would be low in fat and high in nutrients. So these choices would all be good for you.

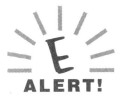

ALERT!

In a society of instant gratification, you are bombarded every day with the next big diet craze. Don't even think about reaching for diet pills or drastically cutting out certain food groups from your diet. These fad diet tricks might produce results initially, but those results don't last, and they don't encourage healthy eating habits. Don't think diet, think nutrition!

When you alter your eating habits to include more plant-based foods and fewer meats and processed foods, you take a powerful step toward improving your health. The best sources of nutrients are minimally processed whole foods, particularly whole grains, vegetables, fruits, and other plant-based foods. These foods are also lowest in concentrations of energy, or in other words, fat.

Getting Ready to Eat Right

How you approach improving your nutritional habits can make all the difference to your success. Keep in mind that a dietary pattern is not a diet. What you need to start thinking about is making a lifestyle shift toward a healthier pattern of eating. This is not a short-term fad diet for quick and easy weight loss. In contrast, this is about learning how to choose a daily diet that is full of nutrient-dense, health-enhancing foods for a longer, healthier, and more enjoyable life that you will share with your spouse and new family.

When you think about nutrition, it's important to realize that as you reduce consumption of some types of foods, you generally increase consumption of other types of foods. So, ultimately, your approach is most successful if you emphasize choosing to eat healthful foods on most occasions, rather than in thinking in terms of forbidden foods, and keep treats that are special and dear to you in your diet. If they happen to be particularly rich and high in fat or sugar, then limit these to very small portions on perhaps one day a week. That way, you feel as if you're enjoying your life and you don't feel deprived.

If you eat a typical fast-food diet, it's challenging to convert to a diet of whole fresh foods. This chapter provides you with specific strategies for making this transition as smooth as possible. Studies show that people are most successful in changing their habits when they focus on the benefits they will receive as a result of their efforts. Your wedding date is a tremendously motivating event for making your *new you* a reality. Keep seeing yourself looking radiant and beautiful in your wedding dress. Put a picture of your dress on your refrigerator door—anything that will help you remind you of how important it is for you to stick to your new commitment.

Adding More Fruits and Vegetables

The first step toward creating a healthy eating pattern is to gradually increase the amount of vegetables, fruits, grains, fish and vegetable oils that you eat and to reduce the amount of meat and high fat dairy products that you consume. Over time, your taste buds will evolve, and you will enjoy more of the subtle flavors of fruits and vegetables. Your meals will be equally tasty, more colorful, and will include more fiber and plant-based nutrients. Not only are you likely to lose weight and feel more energetic, but you're also taking important steps toward reducing your risks of disease, particularly heart disease and cancer.

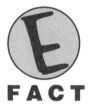

FACT

You might think you're eating okay if you're not eating out or grabbing fast food, but think again. When you're consumed with wedding planning, it's easy to resort to quick, prepackaged foods when cooking. Skip things like instant mashed potatoes or prepackaged noodle dishes. They're high in fat and sodium you don't need. Take extra time, and make things from scratch.

From the fruit and vegetable group, select a variety of fresh foods. Today's frozen and canned vegetables can have as much nutritional value as fresh vegetables. If you're busy, you may be concerned that stocking up on fresh fruits and vegetables is wasteful. Go ahead and buy frozen products. If you buy canned vegetables, either go with a low-sodium variety or rinse the vegetables before serving. Canned fruits should be packed in juice, not syrup.

Another timesaver is packaged, prewashed, presliced vegetables. These are ideal for snacks and salads. They may cost slightly more, but if they help you to incorporate more vegetables into your diet, you will save more in the long run from your health dividends as you age.

Try to brainstorm more ways to add fruits or vegetables at every meal and as snacks during the day. Reduce the amount of meat or chicken in typical combination dishes. For example, in spaghetti, reduce the amount of beef or substitute ground turkey. Then increase the vegetable content in your sauces by adding more mushrooms, bell peppers, celery, or carrots.

Fruit and vegetable juices are also good selections, especially if you can find fresh juices. Be sure the fruit juice you buy is either 100 percent fruit juice or juice and water. Juices can be an excellent source of fruits and vegetables in your diet, *if* you can drink in moderation. One glass of a fruit or vegetable juice is the equivalent of one serving. It's a good idea not to drink more than one glass per day, unless you're very active and burning up lots of energy, because juice has many calories. In addition, it's not as high a source of fiber as the whole fruit or vegetable.

Here are some more tips on how to include more fruits and vegetables in your daily diet:

- At breakfast, slice half a banana or toss some berries or raisins in your cereal.
- Add frozen fruits such as berries or peaches to hot cereals.
- For a mid-morning snack, try carrot and celery sticks with hummus.
- At meals, serve larger portions of vegetables, or prepare multiple vegetable dishes, and have meat as a side dish.
- Prepare meats with fruit toppings or marinades instead of butter.
- Enjoy fruit-based desserts such as poached pears, baked apples, or fresh fruit sorbets.
- Buy packaged prewashed and sliced veggies to pack as snacks or to eat at lunch.
- Eat fresh whole fruits that are in season as snacks or as desserts in the summertime.

- Buy packaged prewashed and chopped fruits to toss into cereals or yogurt or to eat as snacks.
- Add vegetables such as peas or beans into rice or pasta dishes.
- Incorporate multiple vegetables into salads in addition to lettuce.
- Enjoy a smoothie made with fruits or vegetables as a snack.

Keep in mind that all these fruits and vegetables add up to less weight, less disease, less disability, more energy, and a healthy, radiant appearance. Since fruits and vegetables are also rich in fiber, you're likely to feel more full and less likely to indulge in highly processed, high fat, and high sugar snacks.

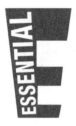

Here's a quick, easy way to add more fiber and vitamins to your diet. If you're a salad eater, switch from iceberg to green, leafy lettuce like Romaine or Boston lettuce. Iceberg lettuce is mostly water, but leafy lettuces are more densely packed with nutritional value. Remember, when it comes to lettuce, the greener the better!

Fruits and vegetables are a great source of fiber, and they contain both soluble and insoluble fiber. Soluble fiber that's part of a healthy diet can reduce blood cholesterol levels and fat absorption. Some fruits and vegetables that contain soluble fiber, in addition to numerous other beneficial nutrients, include apples with peels, oranges, figs, prunes, peas, broccoli, and carrots.

Adding More Whole Grains

Whole-grain foods are minimally processed and therefore rich in vitamins, minerals, and fiber. Grains include whole wheat, brown rice, barley, rye, oatmeal, and corn. Whole grains provide complex carbohydrates that are essential for energy and vitamins A and E, magnesium, calcium, and other important nutrients. These fiber-rich foods contain both soluble and insoluble fiber, but mostly contain insoluble fiber, which aids digestion, keeps your colon healthy, and makes you feel full, helping to prevent overeating and encouraging weight loss.

Processed Grains

In contrast to whole grains, processed grains such as white bread or pasta made from white flour are simple carbohydrates that have lost many of the nutrients and the fiber through processing. These grains are high in sugar (energy or calories) and lower in nutritive value than whole grains. Studies show that eating a lot of processed grains elevates blood fat levels. Read labels carefully to ensure that you're always choosing whole-grain products and not products made from grain parts or enriched grain that has been dyed brown.

Selecting Grain Products

When it comes to grain products, choose products with the word whole in front of the grain ingredient, as well as terms like bran or germ. Sometimes food manufacturers will use enriched flour and dye it a brown color to make it appear like a whole grain. If the ingredient list shows enriched flour as the main ingredient, the grains are highly processed. These are not whole grains, and the product is likely to be high in sugar and low in fiber. Read carefully.

Ideally, eat six servings of grains per day. This may sound like a lot, but a serving size is probably not as large as you may think. Here are some tips to add more whole grains into your daily diet:

- Include a grain-based food at every meal.
- Try whole-grain rolls, breadsticks, and muffins for snacks.
- Purchase whole-grain crackers for meals or snacks.
- Enjoy rice cakes or popcorn that does not include trans fats for snacks.
- Prepare desserts with fruits and whole grains, such as apple crisp.
- Sprinkle wheat germ into your cereal, yogurt, oatmeal, or smoothies.
- Use whole-grain tortillas or pita breads to make healthy chips for dips or salsas.

Because we live in an era of fast food and super-sized products, it's hard to know what a single serving size is. Below is a table with some helpful visual cues.

Food Type	Visual Cue for One Serving Size
fresh fruit	tennis ball
canned fruit	computer mouse
dried fruit	golf ball
fruit as juice	single-serving container of yogurt
fresh vegetables	cereal bowl
cooked vegetables	computer mouse
vegetable juice	school milk carton
sliced bread	CD case
cold cereal	baseball
hot cereal	English muffin
rice or pasta	normal scoop of ice cream

Keep these guidelines in mind when you are making portion choices, and especially try to picture them in comparison with your meal when you go out to eat.

Adding More Healthy Fats and Fish

Consuming fat is not bad in and of itself; unsaturated vegetable fats promote health, while saturated and trans fats undermine your health. Unsaturated fats (monos and polys) are found in plant-based products such as most vegetable oils, nuts, seeds, and whole grains. The one nonplant source of these good fats is deep-water or fatty fish, which are a rich source of polyunsaturated fat. All of these healthy fats play an important role in a nutritious diet.

Fish that come from cold, deep water such as salmon are the best source of healthy fats from fish. The American Heart Association recommends eating fatty fish at least twice a week. More recent information, however, about high mercury levels in fish and high carcinogen levels in farmed fish have caused concern, so be careful about the fish you buy. Wild fish are often safer to eat than farmed fish.

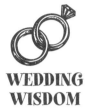

WEDDING WISDOM

It's easy to make the switch to whole-grain bread and brown rice, but what about pasta? If you're a macaroni lover who's loath to give it up, take heart. Many pasta companies are producing whole-grain varieties that include wheat bran, wheat germ, oats, barley, lentils, chickpeas, and flaxseed, making them great sources of fiber, protein, and heart-healthy omega-3 fatty acids.

For good health and weight management, the key is not to eliminate fat, but rather to be selective regarding what *type* of fat you eat—reduce saturated fats, eliminate trans fats, and then replace those fats with unsaturated fats in the diet. Because fats, regardless of their source, are energy dense foods, you should enjoy them in moderation. Here are some tips on how to incorporate unsaturated fats into your daily diet:

- Cook with unsaturated liquid vegetable oils such as olive, canola, or safflower oil.
- Buy tub or liquid margarines with an unsaturated vegetable oil, such as soybean oil, as the first ingredient.
- Sprinkle a few nuts or sesame seeds into your morning cereal.
- Spread natural peanut butter on celery sticks, apples, or green peppers for a healthy snack.
- Dip bread in limited amounts of olive oil instead of spreading it with butter.

Polyunsaturated fats are oils that remain liquid regardless of temperature. Corn, safflower, sunflower, sesame, cottonseed, and soybean oils are all polyunsaturated fats. Deep-water fish also contain polyunsaturated fat that is proven to improve heart health and provide other benefits.

Monounsaturated fats are oils that solidify at cold temperatures. Olive, canola, peanut, most other nuts, and avocado oils are all monounsaturated fats. Foods that contain monounsaturated fats include almonds, cashews, peanuts, and walnuts.

Trans unsaturated fatty acids, often referred to as trans fats, are more harmful to your health than saturated fats. Similar to saturated fats, a direct relationship exists between an increased intake of trans fats and an increase in LDL (bad) cholesterol levels. Additionally, a direct relationship exists between increased consumption of trans-fats and a reduction in HDL (good) levels. Therefore, eating foods high in trans-fats does double damage by increasing your levels of bad cholesterol while simultaneously reducing your levels of good cholesterol.

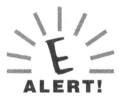

ALERT!

Keep in mind that food manufacturers do not need to list trans fats if the total amount equals 0.5 grams per serving or less. This explains the labels you find that say "no trans fats" and at the same time list hydrogenated vegetable oil on their ingredient list.

Trans-fats are primarily found in commercially processed foods such as pies, doughnuts, cookies, chips, candy, pastries, shortening, and fried fast foods. Food manufacturers create trans fats through a process called hydrogenation that converts otherwise liquid oils into a more solid substance. This hydrogenation is useful to food manufacturers because it increases the shelf life of foods, adds form to otherwise liquid substances, and adds flavor. Studies, however, confirm that there is no level of consumption of trans fats that is considered to be safe to your health and well-being.

Menu Planning for Health

Following your new healthy eating plan requires planning. However, with a minimal amount of organization, you can keep health-enhancing foods in your refrigerator, cupboards, and pantry. Now that you've learned how to include healthier foods in your diet, use these ideas to plan healthy meals. Start using even a handful of these suggestions in your daily life, and before you realize it, you will have shifted to a healthier overall eating pattern.

Breakfast

Breakfast is the most important meal of the day. It's also a wonderful opportunity to eat fiber-rich foods. Plan to include a combination of fiber-rich and protein-rich foods in your breakfast, along with either a fruit or vegetable serving. Great sources of fiber for breakfast include hot or cold cereals and whole-grain breads. Breakfast protein can come from nonfat or low-fat dairy products such as milk or soymilk, or from eggs. You can add fruits or vegetables either by drinking one glass of juice, or by mixing fruit with your cereal dish.

Another great breakfast option is a smoothie. These are easy to make in a blender, with either milk or soymilk, some fruit, and wheat germ or ground flax seed. All of these options can help you start off your day on the right foot.

Lunch

Lunch is another great opportunity to include a rich source of fiber and more fruits and vegetables. Try sandwiches on hearty whole-grain breads with fresh tomatoes, lettuce, and sprouts. For vegetable sources of protein, use bean dips such as hummus on the sandwich. Another option is to use one serving of lean deli meat, like turkey, in a sandwich. Peanut butter is also a great sandwich filling, or you might try avocados.

If packing a lunch, include a vegetable and some fruit. For example, take some prewashed, prepackaged baby carrots or celery sticks. Or slice up a bell pepper into sticks. Easily portable fruits include apples, bananas, oranges, nectarines, grapes, and pears. Try to eat fruits that are fresh and in season.

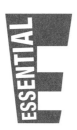

Don't skip meals. Eliminating a lot of calories in one quick swoop is a short-sighted strategy. Your metabolism needs energy frequently and regularly, or else it will slow down and operate as if it's in starvation mode. Instead, eat smaller meals plus a few healthy snacks in between. Then you'll continuously burn energy to your best advantage.

Salads are a great lunch that can be made the night before and can become more filling by adding beans, chickpeas, hard-boiled eggs, or starches such as whole-grain pastas. You can also add grilled chicken, cubes of tofu, or tempeh to your salads for added protein. Tofu can also be added to steamed vegetables, soup, and sauces. Soups are a fantastic source of multiple vegetables and beans. If you combine soups or salad with a hearty whole-grain bread or muffin, you can have a satisfying and nutrient-packed meal. For dessert, try some fresh fruit or poached, baked, or frozen fruits, such as poached pears, baked apples, or fresh fruit sorbets.

Dinner

For dinner, try to shift the emphasis to a vegetable- and grain-based main course with a meat dish on the side. Or, in meals that call for sauces, use a combination of vegetables and meats to reduce the total amount of meat that you consume. For example, you can cut the amount of meat in stew in half and instead add extra carrots, celery, and mushrooms. Try chili with beans and no meat, or use ground turkey instead of beef and add more vegetables instead of meats. Try enjoying stir-fried vegetable dishes with only a small amount of skinless chicken, or simply use tofu instead of any meat product.

Keep in mind that when you eat beans, peas, or lentils together with a dairy product or with grains such as bread or rice, you can obtain the same amount of protein from your meal as if you had consumed a meat dish. Other benefits of eating more beans instead of meat is that they are much more affordable, they contain no saturated fats and no cholesterol, they are nutrient dense, and they are valuable sources of dietary fiber.

If you use canned beans in your foods, try to buy low-sodium varieties and use the liquid that they come packed in for cooking. That liquid is rich in soluble fiber—that's why it has that thick consistency.

Reducing Meat Consumption

You can enjoy meat as part of a nutritious diet. Simply enjoy it in moderation and choose healthy meats. Focus on creating dishes from lean cuts of meats and serving meats as a side dish rather than as a main course. Purchase certified organic meats, also called "free range" meats, rather than commercial meats from animals that have been given an unnatural diet, animal by-products, hormones, and antibiotics. Meat from grass-fed cattle has about one-half to one-third the fat as meat from grain-fed cattle. Grass-fed beef is lower in calories, and higher in vitamin E, omega-3 fatty acids, and conjugated linoleic acid, another health-enhancing fatty acid.

When you prepare meats, try to do so in a manner that reduces rather than increases the amount of fat. For example, baste with wines or marinades instead of animal fat and season with herbs; grill or broil meats instead of frying or breading; sauté or brown meats in pans sprayed with vegetable oils instead of greased with butter. If you are adding meat to other dishes, such as spaghetti sauce, brown it first and pour off the fat before you add it to the sauce. Here are some more preparation tips to reduce saturated fats in meats:

- Trim excess fat from meats.
- Avoid purchasing meats that are marbled with fat.
- Remove skin from poultry.
- Broil, grill, roast, or bake meats on racks that allow fat to drain off.
- Skim fats from tops of stews or casseroles.
- Limit or avoid organ meats, such as livers, brains, sweetbreads, and kidneys.
- Limit or avoid processed meats, such as salami, bologna, pepperoni, or sausage.
- Serve smaller portions of higher-fat meats, such as ham.

These preparation tips not only reduce the harmful saturated fats in your diet, they also lower the total fat that you consume, helping you to manage your weight successfully.

Low or Nonfat Dairy Products

Eating many full-fat dairy products increases the levels of saturated fat in your diet, making it difficult to maintain a lower weight and increasing your risk of heart disease. Dairy products are a valuable source of calcium and protein, but they're not the only sources of these important nutrients. You can still enjoy dairy foods, but be sure to choose nonfat or low-fat versions to promote health.

Cheese, in particular, is a very high-fat food, even higher than beef. While an occasional treat of creamy cheese is not going to harm your overall health, indulging in them regularly will result in stored fat on your body and increase your risks of disease. Here are some practical tips on lowering the amount of saturated dairy fat in your diet:

- Choose nonfat, 1–2 percent, or skim milk, preferably from a certified organic source.
- Select nonfat or low-fat yogurt, sour cream, cottage and cream cheese, preferably organic.
- Use lower fat cheeses for cooking, such as part-skim Mozzarella, ricotta, or Parmesan.
- Enjoy rich, creamy, and hard cheeses on special occasions, not daily.
- Limit the frequency of butter use, and use sparingly.

Check that dairy products come from cows fed grasses and grains rather than meat by-products. Check that milk production has not been accelerated by adding hormones and the cows have been healthy enough not to require constant antibiotics. In addition, look for other sources of calcium in your diet. Vegetables such as broccoli, chard, greens, and artichokes are all great sources of dietary calcium, as well as calcium-fortified orange juice and some whole-grain cereals. Read labels carefully.

Choose Organic

Whenever possible, choose certified organic meats, dairy products, and produce. The reason for this is that large-scale agribusiness producers follow practices that undermine the health value of these foods. For example, these producers give animals large amounts of hormones to accelerate their growth so they can hurry them to slaughter or increase milk production. They feed the animals foods that contain animal by-products to minimize waste, turning otherwise herbivorous animals into carnivores. They feed the animals foods that are not natural to their diets, such as feeding cows corn when they naturally eat grass, which compromises their health and immune systems. To avoid losing these unhealthy animals to illness or death, they give them a constant supply of low-grade antibiotics to increase their resistance to infections.

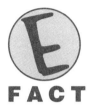

FACT

You've cut back on unhealthy snacks, increased your fruit and veggie intake, and added more whole grains to your diet. So why are you still having trouble losing those extra few pounds? Keep an eye on condiments like salad dressings and mayo, which contain unnecessary fat. Read labels, check the nutritional information, watch serving size, and stick to it.

In contrast, organic farmers allow animals to eat foods that are natural to them. They permit animals to roam freely, to enjoy exercise and fresh air. As a result, these animals produce meats that are lower in levels of saturated or unhealthy fats and higher in health-enhancing fats. These chickens produce eggs that have lower levels of cholesterol. These farmers also use sustainable methods of farming that do not deplete, strip, and destroy the land, but rather support it for continued healthful uses.

The recommendation to eat organic whole grains, fruits, vegetables, and plant-based foods is not meant to be a strict and impossible standard. No one eats a perfect diet. You need to enjoy your life and eating pizza from time to time may be a part of that pleasure. What the recommendation stands for is that the best way to promote your health and well-being through nutrition is to eat a well-balanced fresh, whole foods diet that is rich in plant-based foods, as much as possible. Rely on fast foods and other packaged and processed items as exceptions that are consumed in moderation and do not provide the bulk of your diet.

Healthful Dining Out

With your hectic schedule as your wedding nears, you're likely to be dining out more frequently than usual. Before you buy fast food or order from a restaurant menu, it's a good idea to have a few rules of thumb handy. Today, many healthy choices are available, even at fast food restaurants, which now offer fresh fruit instead of fries, yogurt instead of ice cream or pies, and side salads. When you eat out, stick to the main principles of eating minimally processed, whole, fresh foods and more fruits, vegetables, and whole-grains, and you'll be on the right track.

Portion Control

The main challenge with dining out is that portion sizes are so large. Even if it feels like a bargain, resist the urge to take advantage of larger-sized offerings. When you eat in a restaurant, instead of ordering an appetizer and a main course, order just the main course. Ask the kitchen to divide the portion in half and wrap it for you to take home *before* they serve it to you.

Avoid waiting to eat until you're ravenous. Try to eat slowly to allow your appestat (the part of your brain that controls eating and appetite) to register that you're full. Studies indicate that it takes about twenty minutes for your body to register what you've consumed. Drink plenty of water to help prevent overeating. If you can't resist multiple servings from the bread basket, ask that no bread be served. Or, if it's already on the table, ask for it to be removed.

Hidden Calories

If you drink, enjoy alcohol in moderation. Studies show that one or two alcoholic beverages per day can have a beneficial effect on health. However, watch out for sugary cocktails that are loaded with calories. Instead, choose wine or beer that is rich in antioxidants and other beneficial phytochemicals. Be careful, however, of the loss of inhibition that may come from drinking. Many people tend to overeat after a few drinks. If you fall into that category, you may want to limit your intake until your wedding celebration.

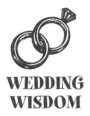

WEDDING WISDOM

Another reason to improve your eating habits is not just fitting into and looking gorgeous in your gown. If you and your husband want children, a healthy diet will be essential when you're pregnant. The sooner you incorporate a healthy and nutritious diet into your daily life, the easier it will be for you to maintain it throughout your marriage.

If once in awhile you splurge, don't beat yourself up. You may need to splurge from time to time and that's okay. It's part of enjoying life. Take it in stride and balance out the extra consumption during the remainder of the week. Make up for it by eating more lightly for a few days and fitting in more physical activity to burn off the extra calories. Avoid all or nothing thinking, and never consider yourself a failure.

Chapter 6

Joining a Gym or Training at Home

Whether you should train at a gym or at home as you're getting ready for your wedding depends on your personal preferences. Ultimately, what's important is that you fit training into your busy schedule. If your budget permits, keep both options open. This gives you the most variety. Training at home is great if you have space because it is the most convenient way to exercise. However, if you need the structure of going to a specific location for your training, joining a club can keep you on track.

Training at the Gym, Home, or Both

Making a commitment to get in shape requires an investment not only of your time, but also of your resources. Before you spend your hard-earned dollars, it's a good idea to consider what is the best way for you to allocate your funds. Certainly, getting in shape does not have to cost a lot of money, nor does it require health club membership. The more options that you have, however, to train and focus on your fitness goals, the more likely it is that you will be successful.

Benefits of Gym Membership

Health club membership provides many benefits besides access to workout equipment. If you choose the right facility, your health club can be like a home away from home.

The following are a few of the benefits that you can expect.

- A safe, supervised environment where CPR, emergency response, and other safeguards are available
- A variety of costly weight and cardiovascular training equipment in a clean and well-maintained setting
- Shower and locker room facilities
- Instruction and support from qualified fitness professionals on program design and exercise execution
- A variety of group exercise classes available on different days and times for convenient training
- Like-minded individuals, new workout buddies, and new friendships
- New activities, exercise styles, or sports that you might not otherwise try
- Services such as child care or other activities especially for children
- Personal training or physical rehabilitation programs
- A place you can always focus on training without interruption, regardless of weather or other circumstances in your life at the time

If the price is right and the location is convenient, joining a health club may be just what you need to stay focused on your fitness program.

Benefits of Training at Home

Training at home is best if you have very little spare time and you have enough space to dedicate to exercising. The primary benefit of training at home is that your home gym space serves as a constant reminder of your commitment to get in your best shape. Access is not a problem because the equipment is in front of you and no travel time is required. Home training cannot be surpassed for ease and efficiency.

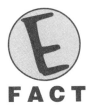

FACT

Fund allocation is all about learning to prioritize so you can get the most bang for your buck. The budget for your exercise program is just one piece of your total wedding budget. Choosing whether to spend on a health club or home equipment will sharpen your prioritizing skills as you weigh up many wedding choices, from food to photographers.

In addition to convenience, another advantage of training at home is that you have plenty of privacy. If you don't like crowds or don't like other people looking at you while you exercise, then home training is for you. Since you're not exposed to the public, you're also not subject to the presence of germs from others, which can be especially terrific during the cold and flu season.

Lastly, if you like being in control of your own environment, you're the master of your own domain. For example, you can adjust the temperature to your liking. If you want to use a fan, you can. If you like listening to music, you can select only the tunes that you want to hear and at the volume that you prefer. If you don't adapt easily to the tastes of others, then home training will give you control over these variables that you cannot control in a gym setting where you must share space with and respect the preferences of others.

Benefits of Gym and Home Training

If funds permit and you can find a good club setting, the ideal situation is to have a gym membership and to train at home as well. This combination gives you the best of both worlds. You have access to all of the club equipment and you can enjoy working out with your friends. For busy days or for days when you want to enjoy privacy, you can squeeze in your training at home.

How to Evaluate a Health Club

If you're considering joining a club, take your time to assess whether it's a good fit for your needs and your lifestyle. In today's market, facilities serve every type of patron. You can train in a women's only facility, in a family-oriented club for people of all ages including children and older adults, or a facility that caters to adults only. Memberships vary depending on how often you want to train and even what time of day you plan to use the club. Doing a little homework before you join can save you from many headaches later.

Types of Facilities

The nature of the community in which you live determines what types of facilities are available. For example, if you live in a major metropolitan center, you'll have many choices. If you live in a less populated location, your choices may be more limited. Keep your eyes open for alternatives other than private clubs.

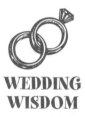

WEDDING WISDOM

Where you live will affect more than just the gym you join. In a highly populated area, you'll have more wedding options, but demand will be high—be prepared to plan far in advance. In a less-populated area, a bit more resourcefulness might be in order when finding services, but with less competition, it's easier to plan in a short time.

The following is a list of some of the many possible alternatives to private health clubs.

- Commercial clubs
- Nonprofit community organizations such as the YMCA, YWCA, or JCC
- College or university campuses with programs open to the community
- Municipal recreation centers
- Hotel or resort clubs or spas that allow local members to join
- Church-based facilities and programs
- Hospital-based wellness centers
- Corporate training facilities

Before you spend any money, find out whether you may already be entitled to some workout perks. Review your health insurance policy and check with your employer to see whether you're entitled to any health club benefits. Many corporations subsidize membership dues or have agreements with facilities for discounted fees for employees. Some health insurance providers also provide sports and fitness club membership benefits.

Touring a Gym

Once you decide on a facility, take a tour at the time of day that you plan to use it. Before you stop by, call and make an appointment. Make sure the hours of operation are going to work for your schedule. Notice how helpful the staff is and whether it's easy to take care of your request. This is your first opportunity to start evaluating the staff and services.

When you arrive, observe all aspects of your experience. Copy the following checklist or keep these points in mind while you enjoy your tour.

- Do you feel welcome when you enter?
- Are the staff friendly, courteous, and helpful?
- Is the facility clean and well maintained?
- Is the fitness staff certified by nationally recognized agencies? Leading organizations to look for include the American Council on Exercise, the National Strength and Conditioning Association, and the American College of Sports Medicine.

- Is the equipment operational and are there plenty of machines available for the number of people who want to use them?
- Is the locker room clean and spacious enough to meet your needs?
- Does the group exercise schedule offer classes that look appropriate for you and at times when you can attend?
- Are the membership fees and requirements flexible enough to meet your needs? For example, some clubs allow you to join on a month-to-month basis; others require an annual commitment with no refund.

If everything meets your needs and the price is right, take at least one day before you sign on the dotted line. Avoid high pressure sales tactics that push you to join immediately. Go home, relax, and think it over. If you feel the same way about it the next day, go back and sign up.

How to Work with a Personal Trainer

While this book provides you with plenty of training advice, if you can afford to supplement your own training with the support of a trainer, it will be money well invested. Even if you only work with a trainer for a couple of sessions to put you through a fitness assessment, to learn how to use equipment, or to critique your form, the information can be very valuable to accelerate your progress.

Reasons to Work with a Personal Trainer

Working with a personal trainer provides several training advantages. A trainer can teach you how to do exercises and critique your form. A trainer can put you through the paces of using equipment so that you feel comfortable when you do your workout. A trainer can customize workouts to satisfy any particular individual needs that you may have. For example, if you have a bad knee or hip and can't do certain movements, a trainer can give you effective alternatives. Trainers also can assess your progress and let you know when it's time to start doing more difficult exercises. Lastly, trainers provide support and motivation to keep you on track.

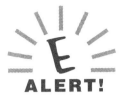

ALERT!

Because you're getting married, hopefully you recognize the importance of being sure before you commit. Do your research before you commit to a facility, whether it is a gym or a reception location. Take tours, chat with staff, and don't be afraid to think things over before you sign on the dotted line. A little research will serve you well.

Studies show that working with a trainer leads to better results in a shorter amount of time. In one study, researchers compared men who did heavy weight lifting over a 12-week period under the supervision of a trainer with those who did the same weight lifting program, but without a trainer. The people who worked with a trainer experienced a significantly greater increase in maximal strength.

Finding the Right Trainer for You

You can use several tried and true methods to find the right trainer for you. Currently, licensing isn't required for personal trainers and local and state governments don't regulate delivery of personal training services. This doesn't mean, however, that your search needs to be a shot in the dark. Reputable certifying organizations exist. These organizations maintain databases of certified trainers and offer locator services.

The National Commission for Certifying Agencies (NCCA) accredits nationally and internationally acknowledged certifying organizations. Accreditation means that the certification processes of these organizations meets standards such as a rigorous and objective examination that is developed to ensure that those who pass meet certain levels of knowledge, skills, and ability, among other criteria. To date, several organizations that certify personal trainers are accredited by the NCCA. These include the following:

- American College of Sports Medicine
- American Council on Exercise
- National Academy of Sports Medicine
- National Strength and Conditioning Association

Contact any of these organizations for referrals for certified personal trainers in your community.

Another great way to find a good personal trainer is through word of month. Positive references from several people you know and trust who have had a good experience with a particular trainer can be very helpful. In addition to getting these referrals, take time to interview a trainer before you start working together. Prepare yourself before you meet the trainer so that you don't waste either your time or the trainer's time. Decide how much money you want to spend and how you want to use the trainer's services. For example, do you just want to have a fitness assessment and introduction to equipment, or do you want to work with someone for several months to guide you through the entire process of your training? You also need to determine whether you want the trainer to come to your home (in which case, you need to have an appropriate space and equipment) or whether you want to work with a trainer at a particular facility.

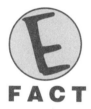

FACT

Trainers have styles that can be loosely characterized as falling into one of the following categories: a drill sergeant who pushes you through your paces; a cheerleader who encourages you with lots of positive motivation; or an entertainer who amuses you. A trainer might even embody parts of each of these styles.

When you've identified what you want the trainer to do for you, then you're ready to interview trainers. Essentially, you want to know whether the particular trainer is qualified to meet your specific needs, whether the trainer's personality and style is a good match for your preferences, and whether the trainer conducts him or herself in a professional manner.

Choosing Group Fitness Classes

Another way to enhance your training program is to attend group fitness classes. The benefits of group classes is that they are more economical than hiring a personal trainer, you can enjoy the fun and camaraderie of working out with others, and the schedule is structured so you can make attending a particular class a part of your weekly routine. The disadvantage of group training is that the exercises are not tailored to your individual needs, but rather the general needs of the group. However, if you select an appropriate class with a group of like-minded individuals that are similar to yourself, you may enjoy the energy of working out with a group and getting the training that you need.

Understanding a Group Fitness Schedule

Today's group fitness schedules feature diversity because clubs cater to a broad variety of participants. To get the best experience, place yourself in the right class for your level and interests. For example, classes are typically divided into beginner, intermediate, and advanced levels. If you're new to exercise or have been exercising for fewer than three months, consider yourself a beginner. Classes also cover the spectrum of fitness categories and include aerobic conditioning, muscle conditioning, stretching, and mind-body exercises such as yoga, Pilates, or tai chi. Many classes offer multiple options, such as cardio-fitness combined with weight training. The key to having a good experience is matching what you want with what is being offered.

Taking Group Cardio and Muscle-Conditioning Classes

Taking group cardio and muscle-conditioning classes is a great way to supplement your overall program. Because getting in shape for your wedding means that your schedule is likely not going to be routine, participating in a group class once a week is a great way to ensure that you always have a backup plan for when you can't do your individualized program. Sample a few classes before you choose one to attend regularly. Different teachers have different styles. You will get the best results in the class where you feel most comfortable.

How to Spot a Good Instructor

Group fitness instructors are certified by nationally recognized certifying organizations. An instructor's main priorities are to ensure the safety of the participants in the class and to provide an effective workout that meets the objectives of the class. This is a tall order. The best instructors are those who make the job look effortless and smoothly lead you from the beginning to the end of the workout. A good instructor also fosters a noncompetitive environment and encourages you to exercise at your own pace. The instructor should provide a variety of exercise options. It's your responsibility to select the one that best fits your body. A good instructor is also approachable. You should feel comfortable asking questions to make sure that you're training at the right level for you.

Creating an Efficient Home Gym

A home gym is ultimately the ideal setting for achieving your workout goals. One of the major barriers to training for people is lack of time. Because stepping into your workout space at home requires no travel time, it's the ultimate in convenience and efficiency. To make it work for you, you simply need to equip it with what you need to achieve your workout objectives and protect your training time and space.

Setting Up Your Workout Space

To set up an effective workout space, you need enough room to move freely. At a minimum, it should be longer and wider than your height. The best situation is if you can set aside space that is always dedicated to your training. If your home, however, does not allow for a dedicated space, then always use the same multi-use portion of your home for training. This space needs to be well ventilated and comfortably temperature controlled. Keep a basket or box for your training equipment so that everything you use will be easy to find and store.

Your workout space can be as elaborate as money can buy or it can be very basic and inexpensive. It all depends on your resources. Your goal is to combine aerobic, muscle conditioning, and flexibility training and to incorporate mind-body exercises. At a minimum, you will need some form of weight-training equipment, which can be as simple as rubber tubing and elastic bands or as elaborate as a weight-training bench and dumbbells. You will need an exercise mat for floor work and a towel or strap that you can use as a stretching tool. If you want to check your form, a full-length mirror is useful.

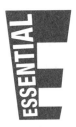

Training safely and effectively requires certain environmental conditions. The ideal temperature for training is between 66 and 70 degrees Fahrenheit, with low humidity. Flooring should absorb impact and should not be slippery. Avoid concrete surfaces and floor rugs. Air should circulate well.`

Protecting Your Training Time

Your most important challenge when you train at home is to protect your training time from interruptions. You need to treat it with the same respect that you would an appointment outside your home. Plan on not answering the telephone or the door, if possible. Turn off your cell phone. Keep pets and other distractions out of the room. Use music to create a positive atmosphere—energizing tunes for when you're working vigorously and relaxing melodies for times when you're winding down. Create a routine so that you use your training space regularly and it becomes part of your weekly routine.

When you train at home, treat it as if you're training at the gym. Wear appropriate exercise attire and athletic shoes. Not only will they protect your equipment and flooring, they will also ensure your comfort and safety.

Buying Your Own Equipment

For the wedding workout, the equipment is simple and affordable. To do the exercises in this book, you will need a good exercise mat, rubber exercise bands or tubing, one or two pairs of dumbbells, and a stability ball. A stretching strap with individualized loops is recommended to improve your flexibility. A sturdy, stable, armless chair is ideal. Be sure that your chair is not on wheels. If you want to buy fancier equipment it's up to you, but it's not essential to be able to do the exercises outlined in this book.

Buying a Mat

A good exercise mat is wide enough to comfortably accommodate your body and long enough to fit your entire body, including your legs. Many types of mats are available in stores. Do not necessarily buy the cheapest mat that you can find because your mat should last many years. Instead, select a quality mat that provides cushioning, support, and is easy to clean and transport. More expensive mats also have antibacterial surfaces, which may not be essential, but are desirable.

Avoid purchasing an ultrathin yoga sticky mat. This will not give you the support that you need for all of your exercises. Avoid mats that are covered with cloth since these are more difficult to clean. Avoid soft foam mats that have too much give because these do not provide sufficient support. A little bit of firmness is desirable with enough give to protect your bones from pressing uncomfortably into the floor.

The ideal, all-purpose mat is a minimum of ⅜" thick and lightweight enough for you to carry easily. Its surface is easy to clean with a sponge. It should have some give but shouldn't completely flatten under pressure so that it provides cushioning between you and the floor underneath. When you train, you can cover it with a towel to enhance cushioning and to absorb sweat.

Selecting Resistance Training Tools

For the muscle-conditioning exercises in this book, you will use your body weight for resistance as in a pushup, or rubber exercise bands or tubing as a tool. If you already own dumbbells, you can use them to increase the difficulty of some of the exercises, but they are not essential. Make sure that you purchase bands or tubing that are specifically designed for exercising. These come in a variety of levels of resistance so you can start at a level that is appropriate for you and progress the difficulty as you become stronger.

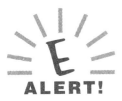

ALERT!

If you have an allergy to latex, you can either purchase latex-free exercise bands and tubing, or you can wear weight training gloves when you work out. Weight training gloves are available in most sporting goods stores and are padded to increase your comfort.

Bands and tubing are fantastic training tools because they are inexpensive—typically costing between five and ten dollars each—and they are lightweight and easy to store. SPRI and Thera-Band manufacture bands that you can buy online or through their catalogs. Fitness Wholesale is a retailer that sells exercise tubing and bands. Look in Appendix D for supplier information.

Buy bands that are at least four feet in length to maximize your exercise options. If you own several bands and tubing, you can store them in a plastic bag with a little bit of baby powder to keep them dry and prevent them from sticking to each other. Check your bands frequently to make sure that they do not have any tears or holes. Replace bands right away when they are worn out, so they don't break when you're using them. Pay particular attention whenever you are using a band around your feet so that it doesn't slip and snap back at you.

Home Cardio-Equipment Choices

For the cardio portion of your wedding workout, you can follow a series of walking workouts at a variety of levels. If you live in an area where you can easily exercise outside, you can do all of these workouts near your home or your office. If you live in an area where weather does not permit outdoor exercise, you can do these workouts on a treadmill at home or at a health club. Alternatively, you can walk at indoor locations such as local malls.

Walking is one of the safest and most effective forms of exercise that requires minimal equipment. All you need is a pair of good walking shoes and appropriate exercise clothing. Studies show that walking as little as thirty minutes on most days of the week can provide health benefits.

Treadmills come in all levels from professional club models that cost thousands of dollars to inexpensive home models that require no electricity and that can be stored under your bed. Before you buy a treadmill, be sure to test it. If you're considering purchasing one from a catalog, make sure that the company permits returns and provides full refunds. Beware of bargains on ultracheap models. Typically, you get what you pay for.

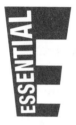

There's more than one "right" way to exercise, and there's no one "right" way to get married. Maybe you'll choose a treadmill at home over a gym membership, and maybe a backyard barbeque beats a fancy reception hall. Whatever your preferences, put your resources toward things that matter most to you.

Other inexpensive ways to get a cardio workout at home include purchasing a step bench and some step workout videos or DVDs. Alternatively, you can purchase a jump rope for quick workouts. If you enjoy exercising to videos or DVDs, a number of high quality products that have been created by fitness professionals are available.

Buying and Caring for Exercise Balls

The only additional pieces of equipment that you will need are two exercise balls, a stability ball and a 5-inch ball you can use as a prop to tone up the inner thighs. Use the table below to make sure that your stability ball is the right size for your body.

Height	Appropriate Exercise Ball Size
Shorter than 4'8"	45 cm ball
Between 4'8" and 5'3"	55 cm ball
Between 5'3" and 6'	65 cm ball
Over 6' tall	75 cm ball

When you sit on your ball, your knees should be at a right angle. A slightly larger angle is okay, but don't buy a ball that is too small. For a softer ball and an easier workout, buy a larger one and underinflate it. For a harder ball and a tougher workout, blow your ball up to full size.

Higher quality balls are burst resistant and deflate slowly. This means that the ball is less likely to puncture, and if it does puncture, it will release air slowly. The worst accidents when using a ball happen when a ball bursts. Buying a higher quality ball with these features reduces the likelihood of this type of accident.

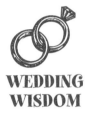

WEDDING WISDOM

Rubber bands, stability balls, and dumbbells might sound like small props, but think of the big results they'll bring. These small props will go a long way when it comes to building your strength, assuredness, posture, and poise as you gracefully glide down the aisle.

You can find a five-inch rubber ball at any toy store. This is a useful prop for when you do your toning exercises to hold between your thighs. Simply gripping the ball requires you to use your inner thigh muscles and will improve their tone. This way you can firm up your inner thighs and slim your legs while you're doing abdominal and other exercises.

Balls are easy to maintain. You can wipe them clean with a damp sponge. Stability balls usually come with a pump. If not, you can find one at a toy or sporting goods store. Because balls leak air, you will need to refill them from time to time. Make sure you keep the floor of your exercise space clean to avoid anything that can puncture your exercise balls.

Chapter 7

Cardio-Fitness— Getting in Peak Shape

Cardiovascular training is a foundation of your fitness program and one of the four basic elements of fitness. Cardio-training, also referred to as aerobics, is your key to successful weight management. Cardio-conditioning exercises burn the most calories, lower your body fat levels, and help you to effectively manage your weight. Having a strong and healthy cardiorespiratory system also reduces your risk of heart disease. This chapter gives you insight into what aerobic exercise is, why it's beneficial, and how much and how hard you need to work to get results.

Aerobic Exercise

Simply put, the term *aerobic* means "with oxygen." When you're doing aerobic exercise, you need to use oxygen to convert your body's stored fat into energy to fuel your body's movements. Activities that are rhythmic, that require moving the large muscles of the lower body, and that are sustained over time are usually aerobic. When you exercise aerobically, you condition your heart, lungs, and circulatory system. You improve your body's ability to draw in, deliver, and use oxygen and to rid itself of carbon dioxide and other byproducts from the energy production process.

Contrary to what you may think, you should not be breathless when exercising aerobically. In fact, during cardio-training, you should be breathing comfortably and be able to speak a few words. Typical activities that are aerobic include walking, jogging, cycling, swimming, and dancing. Even housecleaning can be done aerobically, if you do it with gusto and keep moving continuously.

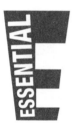

When you exercise aerobically, you elevate your heart rate. The result of regular aerobic training over time, however, is a lower heart rate, both at rest and when you're working. This lower heart rate means that your heart is stronger and working more efficiently.

To improve your aerobic conditioning, you need to regularly stress your body by challenging it to perform continuous rhythmic activities. Aerobic training programs are designed using the elements of frequency, intensity, and time. In other words, you need to determine how often during the week you're going to train, how hard you're going to work when you train, and how long you need to train during each session.

Why Cardio-Fitness Is Important

Enjoying good aerobic conditioning is important because good endurance is essential to having a high quality of life. For example, when you're aerobically fit, you can easily walk up a flight of stairs, you have energy to accomplish daily tasks such as shopping and cleaning, you can enjoy leisure activities such as traveling, sightseeing, and hiking in nature, and you can have fun playing recreational games and sports. If you're planning an active vacation for your honeymoon, it will be all the more enjoyable if you're in good aerobic shape.

In addition to increasing your stamina, if you regularly participate in moderate aerobic activities you will receive many benefits, including the following:

- Lose weight or keep weight at its ideal level
- Reduce body fat
- Decrease appetite
- Tone muscles
- Increase energy
- Keep healthy joints
- Maintain bone density
- Improve depth and quality of sleep
- Improve mood
- Increase feelings of confidence and self-esteem
- Reduce blood pressure
- Lower total cholesterol and increase good cholesterol levels
- Lower disease risks

With all of these benefits, you have many good reasons to get started with your cardio-training program as soon as possible.

Conditioning Your Heart and Lungs

When you exercise aerobically, you specifically condition your heart, lungs, and circulatory system. The ultimate result is a body that works more efficiently at all times, not just when you're exercising. Studies show that after two to ten weeks of consistent training, the heart muscle itself increases in size, resulting in a stronger heart that pumps more blood with each heart beat. Consequently, the heart rate, also referred to as the pulse, is lowered. The volume of blood increases, as well as the amount of hemoglobin that enables the blood to carry more oxygen to working muscles. Regular training also leads to improvements in circulation as more capillaries develop to deliver blood to muscles.

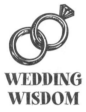

WEDDING WISDOM

Looking for a fun way to kill two birds with one stone in your quest for wedding-planning efficiency? Consider taking dance classes with your fiancé. You'll both get a great cardio workout, and you'll wow everyone at your wedding when you step out at the reception for your first dance.

Regular training improves the body's ability to oxygenate the blood. As the lungs become stronger, they can draw in more air. Another important adaptation to consistent aerobic training is an increase of blood flow to the lungs accompanied by an increase in the amount of lung tissue that can extract oxygen from the air. The net result is that more air is inhaled, more blood is pumped into the lungs, and more oxygen is absorbed into the blood for delivery throughout the body.

Improving Body Composition

Aerobic training is the primary catalyst for reducing your percentage of overall body fat, leading to a better body composition. At the same time that training improves the development of the circulatory system, it also enhances the metabolic system by enabling the body to become more efficient at burning fat for fuel. Studies show that this adaptation can occur after only several weeks of consistent training. The good news is that studies also show that it's not necessary to work at high levels of intensity to become a more efficient fat burner. People have been able to successfully lose fat through short bouts—as little as ten minutes at a time—of cumulative moderate activity.

Other important metabolic changes that come with aerobic training include the more efficient use of sugars circulating in the bloodstream. This is the result of an increased sensitivity to and responsiveness to insulin. Insulin is the key for working muscles to be able to use the sugars circulating in the blood for energy. If you use up the sugars in your bloodstream, they do not end up being converted to fat and stored on your body.

Improve Mood and Well-Being

All forms of exercise, and cardiovascular exercise in particular, improve your mood, increase your feelings of well-being and help to reduce tension and stress. So many studies support the value of exercise for mood improvement that doctors are now recommending exercise as part of a strategy to help or prevent depression. Planning your wedding and getting ready for your married life are among life's most stressful events. Doing regular aerobic exercise will go a long way toward helping you manage this stress and feel good about yourself in the process.

Activities to Improve Cardio-Fitness

Moderate levels of regular aerobic activity improve your level of cardio-fitness. The American College of Sports Medicine (ACSM) recommends that you exercise aerobically at least three to five days a week for twenty to sixty minutes of continuous activity or a minimum of thirty minutes of accumulated activity from short ten-minute bouts. Types of activities recommended by the ACSM include any movement that uses large muscle groups, that can be maintained continuously, and that is rhythmic in nature such as:

- Walking
- Hiking
- Running
- Jogging
- Cycling
- Cross-country skiing
- Aerobic dance or group exercise
- Jumping rope
- Rowing
- Stair climbing
- Swimming
- Endurance games

The U.S. surgeon general defines moderate activity as being roughly equivalent to physical activity that uses approximately 150 calories of energy per day, or 1,000 calories per week. When a task is done at a lower intensity, such as washing a car, you should spend a longer amount of time doing it. For exercises that are done at higher levels of intensity, such as jumping rope, you can spend a shorter amount of time to receive the same benefits. Examples of moderate activity include the following:

- Washing and waxing a car for 45–60 minutes
- Washing windows or floors for 45–60 minutes
- Playing volleyball for 45 minutes
- Playing touch football for 30–45 minutes
- Gardening for 30–45 minutes
- Walking ¾ miles in 35 minutes (20 min/mile)
- Basketball (shooting baskets) for 30 minutes
- Bicycling 5 miles in 30 minutes
- Dancing fast for 30 minutes
- Pushing a stroller 1½ miles in 30 minutes
- Raking leaves for 30 minutes
- Walking 2 miles in 30 minutes (15 min/mile)
- Water aerobics for 30 minutes
- Swimming laps for 20 minutes
- Basketball (playing a game) for 15–20 minutes
- Bicycling 4 miles in 15 minutes
- Jumping rope for 15 minutes
- Running 1½ miles in 15 minutes (10 min/mile)
- Shoveling snow for 15 minutes
- Stair climbing for 15 minutes

The more that you move your body, the more energy is required. For an average sized person, sitting burns approximately 1 calorie per minute, standing burns 2 calories per minute, and slow pacing burns 3 calories per minute. Add more movement into your day at every opportunity.

How Hard to Work—The Training Zone

Studies show that you need to minimally challenge yourself to obtain improvements from your training. For example, if you train fewer than two days per week, at less than 55 percent of your maximum heart rate, or for fewer than ten minutes at a time, you will not get aerobic training benefits. This is not to say that you aren't using energy; rather, what it means is that the level of intensity is not strong enough to strengthen your cardio-respiratory system. Therefore, it's important for you to understand how to monitor how hard you're working, also referred to as the intensity, so that you will know when you're getting a training effect.

Calculating Your Target Heart Rate

You can measure how hard you're working by a variety of methods. One easy way is to calculate your target heart rate. Your heart rate, or pulse, is the number of times that your heart beats per minute. As your workload increases, your heart beats more rapidly and you begin to breathe more heavily. Your heart rate will continue to escalate to a certain point as you near the maximum amount of times that your heart can beat per minute. Then, you must slow down to allow the system to recover. Age and your physical conditioning determine how hard you can work and how long you can sustain a particular level of effort. In general, because the risk of injury increases with intensity and most people don't enjoy working at the limits of their ability, it's better to work at a moderate level.

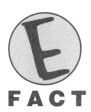

FACT

Newborn infants have a rapid heart rate. A newborn's heart typically beats 220 times per minute. As we age, the maximum rate that our heart beats at slows. This decline is on average a loss of one heartbeat per minute per year of life.

To estimate your training zone, follow these instructions.

1. Subtract your age from 220. This is your estimated maximum heart rate.
2. Multiply your maximum heart rate by 55 percent or by 65 percent depending on whether you are a new or experienced exerciser. New exercisers should use the lower number. This number represents the lower end of your training zone.
3. Multiply your maximum heart rate by 85 percent or 90 percent. Only very experienced and highly fit exercisers should use the 90 percent figure. This number represents the higher end of your training zone.
4. These two figures represent the range of training heart rates for your training zone.

Let's put these figures into practice. Assume that you are a twenty-five year old woman who is new to exercise.

1. $220 - 25 = 195$
2. $195 \times 55\% = 107.25$, rounded to 107
3. $195 \times 85\% = 165.75$, rounded to 166
4. Your training zone = 107 to 166 beats per minute

Using this as a guideline, when you walk, skip, or do any of the other suggested aerobic activities, you want your heart rate to be between 107 to 166 beats per minute. You should be breathing a little harder than usual and breaking a light sweat. You should not be working so hard that you can't talk.

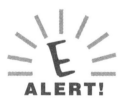

ALERT!

When it comes to smart workouts, the old motto "No pain, no gain" does not apply! Never push yourself to the point of complete exhaustion when exercising. Your goal is to feel good, not sap yourself of all your strength. No one wants to see a limp, listless bride when wedding day rolls around.

The drawback to using this method of calculating your training zone is that it is based on averages and therefore can only provide you with an estimate of what your individualized target zone may be. Depending on your personal history and genetic factors, this estimate may be off by as many as 15 beats per minute. Furthermore, if you're not standing upright while you train, your training zone will also vary. For example, if you're swimming, your heart does not have to work as hard since you're supported by water and you're lying horizontally (your blood does not have to circulate against gravity). In this case, your target heart rate may be as many as 10 to 15 beats per minute lower.

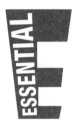

Take your pulse either at your neck or wrist. To take your neck pulse, place two fingers on your temple, outside your eye. Slide your fingers down to your neck until you feel a pulse. Count for ten seconds while keeping your feet moving. Multiply by six.

If you're taking any medications that affect your heart rate, such as those prescribed to regulate blood pressure, your heart rate will not accurately reflect how hard you're working. Pregnancy also affects your heart rate. If you have any medical conditions, be sure to check with your health care provider to determine what an appropriate exercise intensity is for your individual situation.

Using the Karvonen Formula

The Karvonen formula is another method of calculating your target heart rate that is more individualized because it takes into account your resting heart rate. Your resting heart rate is your pulse when you're completely at rest. It's most accurate if it's taken first thing in the morning before you get out of bed. Ideally, to measure your resting heart rate at this time, you should wake up without an alarm, because being startled by a loud clock will elevate your heart rate. Take your pulse for one minute. For further accuracy, take your resting pulse first thing in the morning for several days and use an average of those readings. This is your resting heart rate.

To calculate your training zone using the Karvonen formula, follow these instructions:

1. Subtract your age from 220. This is your maximum heart rate.
2. Subtract your resting heart rate from your maximum heart rate. This number is referred to as your heart rate reserve.
3. Multiply your heart rate reserve by 60 percent.
4. Take this number and add your resting heart rate. The total is the lower end of your training zone.
5. Take your heart rate reserve and multiply by 80 percent.
6. Take this number and add your resting heart rate. The total is the upper end of your training zone.

Let's apply the Karvonen, formula assuming that you are the same twenty-five year old who is new to exercise. Let's assume that you're healthy and your resting heart rate is 75.

1. $220 - 25 = 195$
2. $195 - 75 = 120$ (heart rate reserve)
3. $120 \times 60\% = 72$
4. $72 + 75 = 147$ (the lower end of your training zone)
5. $120 \times 80\% = 96$
6. $96 + 75 = 171$ (the upper end of your training zone)

Using this method, the training zone is between 147 and 171 beats per minute. When you compare the two, you can see that this method allows for a higher heart rate to reflect the individual's good health. At the same time, it is not that much different from the rougher age-based estimate. In general, the Karvonen formula is best for fit people with a history of exercise.

Using a Heart Rate Monitor

The most efficient way to track your heart rate is to use a heart rate monitor. While this is not an essential accessory for training, it's an excellent tool that can teach you a lot about how hard you're working. In addition, you can use your heart rate monitor to measure your resting pulse. Today's models can even store data that you can then upload onto your computer to track over time.

The most accurate heart rate monitors work via a monitor that is strapped to the chest. These are preferable to finger or wrist monitors, because they deliver the most reliable pulse reading. The technology continues to improve and current models are fairly comfortable and unobtrusive.

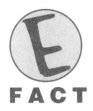

FACT

Heart rate monitors measure your heart rate using a transmitter that straps on to the chest. This transmitter electronically measures the heart rate and sends a wireless signal to a wrist watch that simultaneously displays the heart rate. Some exercise machines have monitors that display heart rate so it's not necessary to wear a wrist watch.

Unless you're interested in collecting data, select a simple model with basic features. The more bells and whistles that a monitor has, the more complex it is to set and the more chances it has to malfunction. Essentially, you need to be able to read your heart rate clearly when you're exercising. Using your heart rate monitor on a regular basis will improve your body awareness. You'll know when you're working aerobically. If you push too hard and become breathless, you'll also see your heart rate elevate. You'll know when to back off to prevent becoming overly winded and having to slow down.

Using Rate of Perceived Exertion

Borg's Rate of Perceived Exertion (RPE) is another easy method of determining your exercise intensity that requires no equipment and is particularly useful if you're taking medications that alter your heart rate. Dr. Gunnar Borg created this scale, also referred to as the Borg Scale. Rate of perceived exertion is based on your subjective evaluation of how hard you feel that you are working. Studies show that this personal estimate is often quite accurate. One caveat is that this scale is most accurate when used during activities that you are familiar with doing. Typically, whenever you learn any new skill, the perception is that it is more difficult and may result in an overestimate of the actual level of exertion.

The original Borg scale used numeric values between 6 and 20, because it was based on studies conducted on twenty-year old college students. The maximum heart rate of 200 represented 220 minus the age of 20 and was represented on the chart as *20*. In subsequent studies Dr. Borg conducted together with his daughter, Elisabeth Borg, they developed a new RPE scale.

Ratings of Perceived Exertion	
RPE	**Subjective Rating**
0	Nothing at all
1	Very weak
2	Weak
3	Moderate
4	
5	Strong
6	
7	Very strong
8	
9	
10	Extremely strong

The Talk Test

The talk test is the least high-tech form of monitoring intensity. Simply put, when you work aerobically, you should not be huffing and puffing breathlessly, but rather breathing at a harder rate than you would be at rest. If you're breathless, it means that you're working at too hard an intensity and you will quickly need to stop, rest, and recover. If you're working at the appropriate aerobic intensity, you are challenging your heart and lungs at a sufficient level to improve conditioning and to continue to train for at least ten consecutive minutes to increase your endurance.

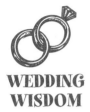

WEDDING WISDOM

If at times you're having trouble fitting in your exercise routine, never lose sight of simple aerobic activities. You might not always have time to hit the weights at the gym or make it to a class, but even fifteen or twenty minutes of walking around your building daily at work will add up to fitness in your wedding-workout crusade.

To gauge this intensity level, the talk test is simple and effective. When you're in your cardiovascular training zone, you should be able to speak a few words and carry on a light conversation. You should not be able to sing or recite lengthy poetry effectively. The talk test is the easiest indicator that you are working at your correct level of exertion.

Frequency and Duration of Your Cardio Workouts

Recall that all training programs are governed by the four variables of frequency, intensity, time, and type. We've just covered the types of exercises that are appropriate for cardiovascular training and the necessary intensity to get a training effect. Now, we're going to look at how frequently you should do aerobic exercises each week and how long your sessions should last in order to gain training benefits.

Defining Your Training Goal

Your individual goals for your aerobic training program determine how often and how long you should train. For example, if you simply want to improve your health and endurance, then you can invest the minimal amount of time necessary to achieve those goals. If one of your training goals includes losing weight, rather than maintaining your current weight, you will need to invest more training time to achieve this result. If you're looking toward improving your competitive performance or participating in races such as 5Ks, 10Ks, half-marathons, or marathons, you will need to invest a considerable amount of time in your training program.

Aerobic Exercise for Health Benefits

To improve your health and reduce your risks of disease, you should train aerobically for at least thirty minutes a day on most days of the week. The good news is that you can still reap benefits from training even if those thirty minutes are accumulated in as short as ten-minute bouts of activity, at least three times a day, for a total of thirty minutes. For example, you can take a brisk ten-minute morning walk, ten-minute lunchtime walk, and ten-minute evening walk for a total of thirty minutes over the course of the day and still meet this minimum standard. For best results, aim to accomplish at least this much activity on a daily basis.

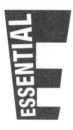

Taking 10,000 steps per day is a good way to measure if you're getting the minimum amount of activity to benefit your health. Studies at the Cooper Institute of Aerobics Research have found that if you wear a pedometer and take 10,000 steps per day, you're likely to have met your minimum physical activity requirements.

You can achieve this much cardio activity by increasing your daily movements. For example, if you drive to work in the morning, park far enough away from your office so that it takes you ten to fifteen minutes to walk there. Use this parking strategy whenever possible, such as when you go shopping or run other errands. This way little walks become part of your daily life. This strategy is efficient because you are constantly adding more exercise into aspects of your daily life and you don't need to carve out big chunks of extra time, which you simply don't have when you're very busy. Studies that compare people who add more movement into each day with people who went to the gym three times a week found that those who added more movement actually burned more calories than the people who went to the gym, but who were otherwise inactive.

Cardio-Fitness for Weight Loss

Increasing the amount of cardio-exercise that you get each day is one of the most effective ways to lose weight, because it burns up lots of energy and requires you to do it over a length of time. Studies show that doing only the minimum amount of exercise to improve your health may not be sufficient if weight loss is your goal. To significantly improve your body composition by ridding yourself of excess fat, you need to move your body for longer periods of time.

Depending on your current level of fitness, you will need to build up your ability to do longer bouts of exercise. Work up gradually to at least one hour a day on most days of the week. If you wear a pedometer to measure your daily steps, aim to walk between 12,000 to 16,000 steps each day. These levels of activity are proven to yield weight loss results when combined with sensible eating habits and effective stress management techniques.

Preventing Injuries

One of the top priorities of your wedding workout shape-up program is to ensure that you avoid injuries. With such an important event coming up, the last thing that you want to do is hurt yourself. Smart training habits go a long way toward preventing injury. Always train conservatively, erring on the side of doing too little, rather than too much.

Signs and symptoms of overdoing it include the following:

- Breathlessness
- Bright red face or very pale face
- Excessive sweating
- Feelings of distress
- Pain
- Dizziness or light-headedness
- Confusion
- Nausea or vomiting
- Pain or tightness in chest
- Racing heart rate
- Feelings of muscle weakness

If you experience any of the above when you're exercising, slow down immediately. Do not resume exercise until you have recovered completely.

Building a Base

The duration of your training sessions when you begin your training depends entirely on your current level of fitness. If you've been completely inactive, you may need to start with as little as ten-minute bouts of activity. If you're already fairly active, then you can start with aerobic sessions as long as thirty minutes or more. The best rule of thumb is to check how you feel both during and after your exercise session. An effective workout leaves you feeling somewhat tired, as though you've worked, but also refreshed. If you feel absolutely worn out, then you have overdone it.

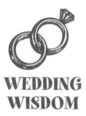

WEDDING WISDOM

Ready to dance the night away on your big day? Your aerobic workouts will get you through the rigors of finishing last-minute errands, like putting together all those programs and favors. They'll also give you an energy boost so you'll stay full of life through your wedding-day festivities—morning to midnight. Your flowers will wilt long before you do!

Once you determine the length of your sessions to begin with, you need to build a base of endurance activity before you progress to significantly longer sessions. For example, if you're doing daily walks of thirty minutes on a regular basis, it's not a good idea to suddenly increase this level of activity to one hour walks. Instead, build your conditioning level up gradually over time. Starting your conditioning program well in advance of your upcoming marriage provides you with the time you'll need to gradually increase your activity levels.

How to Progress

In general, increase your amount of cardiovascular training by no more than 10 percent per week. If you find that you are feeling overly tired or sore, than scale it back and increase by only 5 percent. Here's an example to apply this principle. If you're walking thirty minutes a day, five days of the week, increase this amount to thirty-three minutes a day, five days of the week, or add up to fifteen more minutes over the week on individual days for a thirty-five minute walk three days a week and thirty minute walks on two days of the week. Stick with this new program for at least two weeks before you increase it again. When you start incorporating longer aerobic exercise sessions of more than forty-five minutes in length into your program, be sure to rest at least one day per week.

Chapter 8

Weight Training—Building Strong and Toned Muscles

Weight training, also referred to as resistance training, is a critical component of your wedding workout program to improve your well-being and to provide tone and definition to your physique. Weight training builds valuable muscle mass that increases your endurance and energy levels, prevents injuries, helps you burn more calories to reduce body fat, and improves your sense of control over your body. This chapter helps you understand what weight training is, why weight training is beneficial, and how much and how hard you need to work to get results.

Introduction to Weight Training

Weight training enables you to strengthen your muscles and build muscular endurance through exercises that challenge your major muscle groups to work harder, thus stimulating them over time to become stronger and to develop more endurance. This conditioning process improves the neuromuscular connectivity of your mind and body and builds muscle tissue. Weight training uses many forms of resistance including weight machines, free weights, elastic tubing and bands, or body weight. Resistance training conditions your muscles and the connective tissue that includes your tendons and ligaments, and strengthens your bones. As you become stronger, your energy level and your ability to do physical work increases.

Your Major Muscle Groups

A well-balanced resistance training program includes exercises for all of your major muscle groups. The major muscle groups of your body include the following:

- Chest
- Back
- Shoulders
- Front of upper arm
- Rear of upper arm
- Buttocks
- Front thighs
- Rear thighs
- Calves
- Abdominals

Your workout needs to include at least one exercise for each of these major muscle groups to create balanced muscle development. Muscles exist in opposing groups and work together synergistically. The biceps (the muscle in the front of your upper arm) and triceps (the muscle in the rear of your upper arm) is an example of a muscle pair. When the biceps contracts and shortens, the elbow bends and the triceps lengthens. When the triceps contracts and shortens, the arm straightens and the biceps lengthens. Well-balanced muscles support joints and improve stability. Lack of balance in muscular development contributes to poor posture, unstable joints, and an increased risk of aches, pains, and injury.

Muscle Function: Movers and Stabilizers

Your skeletal muscles provide two basic functions: movement and stability. The muscles and skeleton give the body structure, form, and the ability to move. For example, when you walk and take a step, you're using many muscles, including several muscles of the lower body: the muscles of your calves, thighs, hips, and buttocks. At the same time that these larger muscles are enabling you to move, other muscles are supporting your spinal column and hips, making sure that you keep your balance and move efficiently. Most of the "mover" muscles of the body are closer to the surface, while the "stabilizer" muscles lie deeper within, closer to the spinal column. Some muscles function as both movers and stabilizers depending on the particular action of the body.

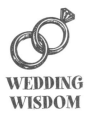

WEDDING WISDOM

Start pumping those muscles up now, before you get married, because you'll need plenty of muscle strength as you and your husband begin your new married life together. If you're moving into a new place, think of all the boxes you'll be lugging around!

The function of specific muscles is relevant when it's time to decide whether the goal of your training is to improve strength or endurance. Most mover muscles need a combination of strength and endurance. In contrast, stabilizer muscles primarily need high levels of endurance conditioning to function at their best.

Why Resistance Training Is Important

Resistance training is important because we need strength and endurance to enjoy everyday living, and the comforts of modern living have removed most of the natural physical challenges from our lives. For example, if we lived in a state of nature, we would need to hunt and gather our food, prepare it, build and maintain our shelters, create our clothing, and so on. Historically, these tasks required manual labor. Modern American living, however, requires very little physical work. Most of us need to strategically incorporate physical challenges back into our lives in order to keep our bodies healthy and our muscles strong. Accordingly, weight training is a necessity of contemporary living if you want to be at your best.

Consistent weight training provides the following benefits:

- More strength and endurance
- Increased self-confidence
- Better posture and balance
- Toned and healthy appearance
- Less likelihood of injury
- Lessen or eliminate back pain
- Stronger bones
- Healthy joints
- Better depth and quality of sleep
- Less stress
- More muscle mass and less body fat
- Higher metabolism
- Lower blood pressure
- Lower LDL (bad) cholesterol and total cholesterol levels
- Lower risks of disease such as heart disease and diabetes

You can see from all of these benefits that getting into the habit of weight training not only boosts your confidence and adds definition to your figure for your wedding, it starts you on the path to healthier, more active living during your married life.

Enjoying Life Fully

Regular resistance training improves musculoskeletal health so that you can complete all of the tasks that you need to with vigor and enthusiasm. In addition, people who have more muscular strength and endurance in the younger adult years are more likely to enjoy independent living as they age. Fifty percent of adults over the age of forty cannot carry a ten-pound bag of groceries, according to the National Center for Health Statistics. Keeping your muscles strong and healthy gives you more energy to complete your household tasks such as grocery shopping or visits to the florist. This extra energy will serve you well as you run the numerous errands you need to organize your upcoming wedding.

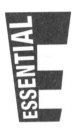

Strength training is not just for chores at home. If you like to bring everything short of the kitchen sink on vacation, strong muscles are your ticket to packing freedom. Pack all you want—you'll be strong enough to tote your luggage everywhere yourself! Just don't pack over the airline's suitcase weight limit.

Improving Body Composition

Most people think of aerobic exercise as the key to improving body composition, but resistance training also plays an important role in creating a lean physique because it helps you to build and retain lean muscle mass. Maintaining a good ratio of muscle mass to fat mass does more than improve appearance. It is a key health factor. After the age of thirty, people begin to lose muscle mass unless they actively work to keep it. The average loss of muscle is approximately ⅓ to ½ pound per year. At the same time, the average person gains one to two pounds of fat per year. The typical person, therefore, gradually becomes fatter and weaker over time. This cycle of weight gain, muscle loss, and loss of abilities can be avoided with weight training.

Studies show that the most effective programs for losing weight and keeping it off combine aerobic exercise, resistance training, and healthy nutritional habits. People who followed programs that included all three components were more successful with their weight loss and management goals, when compared to people who tried to diet alone, or to people who only added aerobic exercise in combination with new eating habits. If weight loss is part of your goal for the wedding, do not skip weight training.

Building and Keeping Strong Bones

Studies confirm that weight training is the best way to build and maintain strong, dense bones. For women in particular, it's important to build dense bones when young up to age thirty and to avoid the loss of bone mass after age thirty. After menopause, women are at particular risk of osteopenia or osteoporosis, a bone thinning disease.

The American College of Sports Medicine has issued a position on Bone Health with recommendations for exercises that preserve bone. The recommended strategy is to do a combination of weight bearing aerobic activities such as stair climbing, walking, jogging or jumping, and resistance training.

Improving Self-Confidence

Resistance training also improves your self-confidence because as you improve your physical abilities, you feel better about yourself and you have a stronger sense of control over your own environment. This confidence can be a real boost when you're struggling with all of the challenges that a wedding can bring. Overcoming some of your own personal limitations and discovering how strong you can become is exciting and rewarding. For women in particular, who tend to be weaker in the upper body, building strength and being able to lift and carry things, and load up your own bags and suitcases can feel very empowering.

Understanding Key Resistance Training Principles

Now that you realize all the benefits weight training brings to your life, you need to understand key resistance training principles to get started with your program. Once you comprehend these principles, your training becomes much more meaningful. Rather than simply going through the motions, you understand why you're doing the number of reps, sets, and exercises that you follow in your program. Here's a brief overview of all the essential concepts that you need to master.

- **Strength:** Muscular strength is the maximum amount of weight that you can lift at a single time, known as your one-rep max. To improve strength, use heavy weights and do few reps. Strength training tends to build larger-sized muscles.
- **Endurance:** Muscular endurance is the number of times that you can lift a sub-maximal weight over time before you can no longer lift it again. To improve endurance, use lighter weights and do more reps. Endurance training tends to build longer, leaner muscles.
- **Overload:** To improve strength or endurance, you need to challenge your muscles or "overload" them to do more than what they usually do.
- **Failure:** To achieve overload, you need to take your muscles to "failure." When your muscle reaches failure, you cannot do one more rep of that particular exercise with perfect form.
- **Rest and Recovery:** After your muscle experiences failure, it must "rest and recover" before it can do more work. Rest refers to the time in between sets, as well as the time in between workouts. For strength training, rest periods are longer between sets than for endurance training.
- **Specificity:** Muscles develop "specifically" in response to how they are trained. For example, if you emphasize strength training, muscles will become stronger. Muscles become conditioned through the "SAID" principle: Specific Adaptation to Imposed Demand.

- **Reps:** A repetition or "rep" is one completely executed exercise movement. For example, one pushup is one rep.
- **Sets:** A set is a group of consecutive reps that you do without resting. In other words, when you do the last rep of your set, your muscle has reached failure.
- **Workout:** A workout is an organized training session composed of particular exercises, reps, sets, rest periods between sets, and a specific exercise order.
- **Progression:** As your muscles respond to overload and become stronger and increase their endurance, you need to progress or advance your program to continue to experience overload. This is referred to as progression. Always progress conservatively to avoid injury.

The frequency, duration, and intensity of your weight training refers to how many days per week you need to train, how long you need to train during each session, and how hard you need to train to achieve your desired results. These aspects of your training program depend on your goals. For example, a program to build strength emphasizes fewer sets and heavy weight loads. A program to increase muscular endurance focuses on multiple sets of high numbers of repetition and lower weight loads. If you want to achieve a combination of strength and endurance, your program would feature a mix.

Defining Your Training Goals

For purposes of the wedding workout, your program is based on improving health and accordingly your appearance as a vision of health and radiance as you walk down the wedding aisle. The American College of Sports Medicine recommends the following guidelines for beginning a muscular strength and endurance training program for young, healthy adults:

- For each exercise, perform 1 set of 8 to 12 repetitions.
- Perform 8 to 10 different exercises per workout, covering all major muscle groups: arms, shoulders, chest, abdomen, back, hips, and legs.
- Train with weights 2 to 3 days per week, taking a day off in between workouts.

Stick with this basic conditioning program consistently for a minimum of two months before trying any more advanced training techniques. After you have established this basic level of conditioning, you can start using other program modifications if you want to build more muscle definition or power or simply to add variety and keep it interesting.

Understanding Your Body Type

Before beginning your training program, it's good to understand your body type because you can approach your training slightly differently or modify your program according to your body type to get your ideal results.

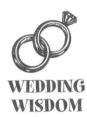

WEDDING WISDOM

If you have a sleeveless or strapless gown, your look is sure to be striking and streamlined. But those dress styles also mean your arms are front and center—and you don't want flabby arms to go with your fabulous dress. Weight training is the way to go to sculpt shapely arms and give yourself great muscle definition.

For classification purposes, body types are divided into three main categories: ectomorph, mesomorph, and endomorph. These body type characteristics are genetic and represent your personal heritage from your family tree. You do not have any control or choice in the matter, just as you cannot alter your height or the natural color of your hair or eyes. Most people are a combination of types with one particular aspect that plays a more dominant role. Each of these body types responds somewhat differently to training.

Ectomorph

The ectomorph is the typical delicate small-boned, lean person. The ectomorph usually has a difficult time adding muscle mass to her body and is most challenged by weight training. It's very difficult for an ectomorph to get "big" from weight training. In fact, ectomorphs do not put on weight easily. The ectomorph tends toward more "slow twitch" muscle fibers that are naturally designed for muscular endurance. Therefore, the ectomorph usually enjoys and is good at aerobic training and needs to make a real commitment to fit weight training into her schedule.

Endomorph

The endomorph is the typical large-boned, full-figured, curvaceous person. Most endomorphs have a pear-shaped figure, larger in the hips than in the upper body. The endomorph usually has a lot of natural strength and is good at weight training. In fact, the endomorph may be able to build muscles that are larger than she would prefer and may want to emphasize endurance, rather than strength training. The endomorph typically does not enjoy aerobic training and gains weight easily. In contrast to the ectomorph, the endomorph needs to make a strong commitment to fit aerobic training into her schedule.

Mesomorph

The mesomorph is the typical medium-boned, muscularly built person. The mesomorph is in-between the other two body types and has an athletic appearance. The mesomorph can build muscle size and definition more easily than either the ecto or the endo. The mesomorph is better at weight training than cardio training and can build muscular strength and power that is essential for speed and short bursts of high energy. The mesomorph is well-balanced and needs to make a commitment to keep up with a balanced training program.

Keep in mind that most people do not fit absolutely into one category. It is useful to understand these general principles, however, so that you can determine where you fall in the spectrum and consider what you may need to emphasize in your own training. The best conditioning program is not a one-size-fits-all, but rather, is tailored to your own unique requirements.

Frequency and Length of Workouts

For optimal muscle conditioning results in your wedding workout program, train your total body three times a week. In between workouts, allow forty-eight hours of rest for muscles to repair and recover. For example, you could plan to weight train on Mondays, Wednesdays, and Fridays. Seventy-five percent of your conditioning benefits come from a minimum of two workouts per week. Therefore, if you're busy, make a minimum commitment to train each of your major muscle groups two times a week to achieve and maintain physical improvements. If you want to get results more quickly, stick with a training schedule of three times per week.

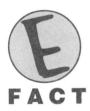

FACT

To manage back pain or injuries, you need both strong back and stomach muscles. Weight training and strengthening exercises aimed at the back and stomach help to build stability and keep everything in alignment.

Research shows that you can get effective training results with as little as one set of an exercise for each of the major muscle groups of your body. Since you have ten major muscle groups, the minimum amount of exercise that you need to do to improve your health is only ten sets. This can be accomplished in fewer than twenty-five minutes. Of course, this is a minimum. If you want more visible and rapid results, you need to invest more time. The good news is that when you're very busy, you can squeeze in only a few exercises and still gain some benefits. Something, even a short ten-minute workout, is better than no exercise at all.

Weight Training for Toning and Shaping

To achieve visible toning results, ideally you should follow a program that includes at least three sets of an exercise for each of your major muscle groups. Rather than doing three sets of the exact same exercise, try challenging your muscles in a variety of ways by doing a different targeted exercise for each muscle group. For example, instead of doing three sets of triceps dips, do one set of triceps dips, one set of triceps pushups, and one set of a reverse plank. Each of these exercises challenges your triceps muscle, but in a slightly different manner. Doing all three of them in one workout maximizes the number of muscle fibers that you can work.

Depending on your current level of fitness, you will need to build up the ability to do three sets of an exercise for a specific muscle group. Work up gradually by doing a program of one-set training for the first six to eight weeks. After the first two months of basic conditioning are complete, start adding in more sets to really start targeting your muscular development.

Intensity: Selecting the Right Resistance Level

When you begin your training, you want to start at a lower intensity level and focus on proper form. To get the best results from your training, you want to achieve muscular failure by the last rep of your set. Begin training safely with a repetition range of ten to twelve. If that feels like too much for you, go ahead and do as many as twelve to fifteen reps with a lighter weight to muscle failure.

Beginning with a lighter load decreases your risk of injury. This early phase of training gives your joints, ligaments, and tendons a chance to become conditioned as your muscles get stronger. You can also focus more on learning the exercises and doing each repetition correctly. Add weight gradually once you feel confident with your technique.

The weight load or level of resistance that you choose determines the number of reps that you can do. The best way to find a proper weight level for you is initially through trial and error. Always start out on the conservative side with a weight you think might be light for you, or if you're using an elastic band or tubing, with a lightweight resistance level. If you can lift a weight or do an exercise easily for fifteen repetitions, the resistance is too light. Increase the weight, or if you're using bands or tubing, either combine two lightweight pieces together or use a heavier weight band or tubing, so that the last couple of reps feel difficult and the muscle is fatigued. Ideally, you should be able to perform one set of eight to twelve reps in about fifty to seventy seconds, or approximately one minute.

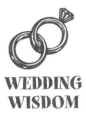

WEDDING WISDOM

Any exercise that gets you in shape *and* boosts your metabolism is a double winner! There will be tons of great food to eat at your wedding, not to mention on your honeymoon. Instead of depriving yourself during these wonderful times, earn the chance to splurge, knowing your metabolism is doing its best for you because of your workouts.

The number of reps per set that you do indicates the intensity level. When you are working in a twelve to fifteen rep range to fatigue, you're working at approximately 65 to 70 percent of your one max rep. The following calculations show how hard you are working at a particular rep range. One repetition represents the absolute maximum amount of weight that you can lift with the particular muscle group that you are challenging.

- 1 rep = 100%
- 2–3 reps = 95%
- 4–5 reps = 90%
- 6–7 reps = 85%
- 8–9 reps = 80%
- 10–11 reps = 75%
- 12–13 reps = 70%
- 14–15 reps = 65%
- 16–20 reps = 60%

It's always more difficult to work at a higher level of intensity. And, when you work at higher intensities, you increase your risk of injury. At the same time, if you don't work hard enough, you are not going to receive training benefits. To achieve results, your efforts need to be at least 65 percent.

As you advance your program and begin working at heavier levels of resistance, progress gradually. When you start out at a new resistance level, you want to begin at the lower end of the rep range and work your way up by increasing the number of the reps before you increase the weight level. This is a more conservative approach that reduces your risk of injury.

Progressing Your Program

In addition to working at the right intensity level, progressing your program properly will prevent injuries and ensure effective results. After six to eight weeks, you can add to your program by increasing the number of sets (up to three sets) or by increasing the amount of weight (up to 5 percent). This weight increase should be to the point where you cannot perform more than twelve reps before your muscle is fatigued. Remember, muscles require approximately six to eight weeks to adapt to a new program.

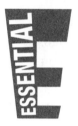

Unless you are training to be a body-building champion, your weight-training routine will probably focus more on endurance. You won't need muscles bursting your wedding dress at the seams. Longer, leaner muscles will fit any wedding look perfectly.

Fewer reps means that you are using a heavier weight. For example, a typical progression may be to perform one set of eight reps. As you become stronger, you can increase to one set of ten reps, all the way up to twelve reps. After you have achieved the ability to lift that weight with good form twelve times, you can either add one or two more sets. Alternatively, you can increase the challenge by increasing the weight so that you are once again lifting one set of eight reps to fatigue.

Training Tips for Effectiveness and Safety

Before you lift that first weight, you need to review basic guidelines and techniques to keep your training safe and effective. Follow these basic tips and soon you'll be looking and feeling great.

Always warm up for five to eight minutes before you start any strength or toning exercises. Any rhythmic activity that uses the large muscle groups of the hips and legs—like walking, marching or jogging in place, jumping rope, or riding an exercise bicycle—provides an effective warm up. The warm up increases blood circulation to the muscles, stimulates smooth movement in the joints, and prepares the body and mind for physical effort.

Always remember to breathe. Holding your breath can elevate blood pressure. If you find yourself holding your breath or breathing in short spurts, check your breathing periodically during the workout and cool down.

With every exercise, begin with good posture. This position supports the natural curves of your spine and can be identified by imagining a plumb line through your body, with your head above your shoulders, shoulders above hips, hips over knees, knees over ankles, and feet pointing forward. Tighten your abdominals to provide support to your lower back. Since physical tension can inhibit smooth, efficient movement, consciously release excess tension throughout your body, especially in your shoulders.

When you use any handheld equipment, keep a solid yet relaxed grip. Avoid squeezing your weights because it can elevate blood pressure. Tubing generally comes with handles and should also be held with a relaxed grip. For bands, you can secure the end between your thumb and index finger and make a fist. To increase hand comfort, wear padded weight training gloves.

Use slow, controlled, rhythmic movements. Proceed through a full range of motion with each rep and hold the exercise position for a moment at the peak muscular contraction to ensure that you are fully stimulating the targeted muscle fibers. Avoid swinging weights or using momentum. Feel the exercise in your working muscles. Be careful not to strain your joints.

Choose at least one exercise for each muscle group. Use a variety of resistance techniques—weights, bands, tubing, body weight—to challenge your muscles in different ways for better results.

In general, training your largest muscle groups before smaller ones will lead to optimal results. For example, muscles can be trained in the following order:

1. Hips and legs
2. Chest and back
3. Arms and shoulders
4. Abdominals and back

Core training comes last because core stabilizers are necessary to stabilize your body during the workout, so you don't want to exhaust them early in the workout.

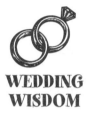

WEDDING WISDOM

Did your seamstress hit a snag in your alterations? Can't make your seating arrangement work? Keep your cool by breathing deeply. It's tempting during a tough workout or a stressful situation to take short, shallow breaths, but catch yourself! Good breathing techniques are handy for more than just your training sessions.

The cool down can consist of stretches for the targeted muscle performed at the end of each set or a series of stretches performed at the conclusion of your workout. Either method prevents muscle soreness and enhances conditioning benefits.

Remember:

- Warm up
- Breathe
- Maintain good posture
- Avoid excessive gripping
- Use proper form
- Exercise choice
- Exercise order
- Cool down

The most important reason for using correct training techniques is injury prevention. Keep these points in mind every time that you train and you'll be radiant and healthy for your wedding date.

Avoiding Overtraining

One of the risks of getting excited about your training program is trying to do too much, too hard, too soon. With your wedding coming up, the last thing that you want to do is undermine your health by overtraining. The American College of Sports Medicine has a comment paper titled "Overtraining with Resistance Exercise" that explains causes, signs, and symptoms. Avoid overtraining by progressing your program safely and sensibly.

Causes of overtraining include the following:

- Training too many times a week
- Doing too many exercises per session
- Lifting too many sets
- Consistently lifting overly heavy weights

Signs and symptoms of overtraining include the following:

- Strength loss
- Chronic fatigue
- Poor sleep
- Appetite loss
- Excessively sore muscles
- Mood changes
- Loss of interest in training
- Increased frequency of illness with slower recovery

If you recognize any of these symptoms, take a look at your program and modify it to include more rest and recovery and a lower intensity.

Use the following strategies to prevent overtraining:

- Progress your program as outlined
- Avoid repetitive training (training with no variety)
- Avoid straining muscles or joints through overuse
- Combine your weight training with aerobic, stretching, and mind-body exercises

Because you're likely to be so busy planning your wedding, the odds of overtraining are slim. However, because it does happen to some people, it's worth understanding, if only to give you a good appreciation of the importance of rest, recovery, and variety in your program.

Chapter 9

Weight Training— Upper Body Exercises

A strong and toned upper body is important to improve the quality of your daily living and to improve your appearance, particularly in a wedding gown. Most women are very weak in these muscles because day-to-day activities require little upper body strength. By doing these weight training exercises regularly, you'll notice that you're more able to lift and carry things comfortably and that you'll have healthy looking, toned shoulders, arms, and a toned back to show off in your wedding dress.

Training Your Chest

All of the following exercises (in the chest training section and in the sections that follow) can be done at home or at the gym, whatever works best for your schedule. You can use dumbbells or bands and tubing and body weight to achieve the desired level of challenge. Whenever possible, each exercise presents multiple variations so that you can diversify your workouts over time and use whatever equipment that you have available.

Developing your chest muscles is important to provide necessary support for your breasts and to maintain strong and healthy shoulder joints. Most people have tight chest muscles, so a thorough program of stretching and opening up your chest area is important to balance any additional training. Enjoy the rewards of your hard work with more defined cleavage and perkier, uplifted breasts as you stroll down the aisle in your wedding gown.

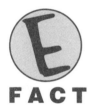

FACT

Since most women are weaker on top with stronger muscles in their lower bodies, you can use these upper-body exercises to help balance things out. If you're feeling a bit bottom heavy when you try on your wedding dress, these exercises will help to bring some attention upward.

You use your chest muscles on a daily basis. Any movement that involves pushing something away from you with your arms uses these muscles. Any big hugging motion also involves these muscles. These common actions, however, are not conducted with sufficient resistance to challenge your muscular strength or endurance. Therefore, supplemental weight training is necessary to maintain the health and tone of these important muscles.

Your chest muscles are layered and include the pectoralis major and the pectoralis minor, known collectively as the "pecs." The pectoralis major is a large fan-shaped muscle that is closer to the surface. Part of the pectoralis major attaches to the middle of the collarbone and runs to the upper arm in a horizontal direction. The pectoralis major works together with your shoulder muscles to move your arms forward, upward, across the front of your body, and to rotate your arms inward.

The other part of the pectoralis major runs from the sternum, or breast-bone, in the center of your chest across your chest and up to the top of your upper arm in a diagonal direction. When you press your arms downward and inward you contract these muscles. Training on an incline bench will enable you to most effectively challenge these muscle fibers.

INCLINE CHEST PRESS

Figures 9-1 and 9-2

The incline chest press tones and strengthens your chest, shoulders, and arms. It also tones the muscles that provide lift and support to the breasts.

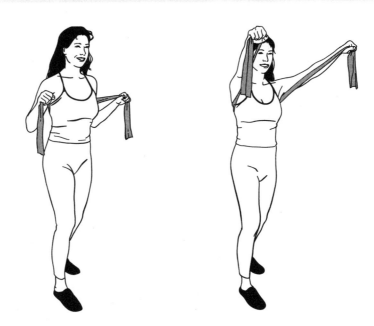

GET SET Stand in a split stance with your feet hip-width apart and one foot slightly in front of the other. Hold one end of an exercise band or tubing in each hand with the band or tubing behind your upper back. Hold your hands at chest height without hunching your shoulders with your palms facing downward. Pull in your abdominal muscles to support your lower back. (**SEE FIGURE 9-1.**)

ACTION Slide your shoulders down and back. Press your arms up at a forty-five degree angle, keeping your palms facing downward, without locking your elbows. Feel all your chest muscles contracting, particularly in the upper central area. Keep your shoulders relaxed, abdominals pulled inward. Keep your wrist joint flat. (**SEE FIGURE 9-2**).

WEDDING WORKOUT POINTERS Inhale to prepare, exhale as you press up. Inhale, return to start. Avoid arching your lower back by contracting your abdominals and pulling your lower ribs in toward your spine. Lengthen arms without locking elbows.

VARIATIONS

(EASIER) Lie on top of a band or piece of tubing behind your back. Hold one handle in each hand. Bend knees with feet flat on ground. Press rib cage into the ground using abdominal muscles. Press up against resistance. Lower slowly.

If you experience any discomfort in your elbows or shoulder, do not lower weights all the way back to start. Try lowering only partially down and keep weights above shoulders.

(HARDER) Use dumbbells and sit on an incline bench with your feet flat on the ground. Make sure your lower back is supported against the bench. Exhale as you push weights up and away from body. Inhale as you return to start.

CHEST FLY

Figures 9-3 and 9-4
The chest fly tones and strengthens your chest and shoulders. It also provides definition to your cleavage.

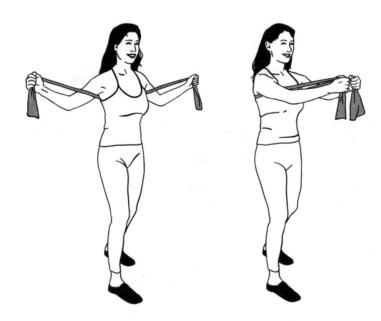

GET SET Stand in a split stance with your feet hip-width apart and one foot slightly in front of the other. Hold one end of an exercise band or tubing in each hand with the band or tubing behind your upper back. Hold your arms fully extended out wide at chest height with your palms facing inward without locking your elbows or hunching your shoulders. Pull in your abdominal muscles to support your lower back. (**SEE FIGURE 9-3**.)

ACTION Slide shoulders down and back. Bring your arms toward each other in a big hugging motion. Feel your chest muscles contract, particularly in the center. (**SEE FIGURE 9-4**.)

WEDDING WORKOUT POINTERS Inhale as you open your arms, exhale as you hug and squeeze.

VARIATIONS

(EASIER) Lie down on top of a piece of tubing behind your back. Hold one handle in each hand. Start with both hands extended outward with elbows slightly bent. Make a big hugging motion against resistance. Lower slowly.

(HARDER) Perform this exercise on an incline bench while holding a dumbbell in each hand. Place your feet flat on the ground. Maintain good alignment. Hold weights with your palms toward each other. Push dumbbells over chest with arms fully extended without locking elbows. Slowly, lower arms outward until arms are parallel with the bench. Lift arms back to start in a big hugging motion. Avoid any feelings of strain or discomfort in the shoulder joint.

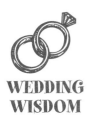

WEDDING WISDOM

Forget padding the top of your dress for extra cleavage! Focus on exercises like the incline chest press and chest fly—if you have a strapless, sweetheart, or other open-neckline dress, these are the exercises for you. They won't magically increase your bust size, but by improving definition and adding a little lift, you'll achieve a more flattering look.

PUSHUP

Figures 9-5 and 9-6

Pushups tone and strengthen your arms, shoulders, and chest. They also challenge your core muscles to support good posture.

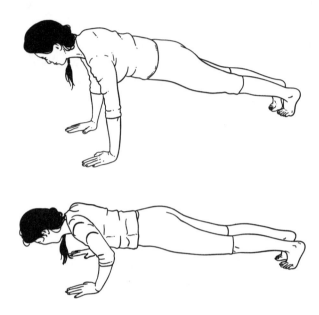

GET SET Kneel on all fours on the floor. Walk your hands forward until your hands are slightly wider than shoulder-width apart and your torso resembles a slanted board. Tighten your abdominal and buttock muscles to support your lower back. Maintain good alignment. Lift the tops of your feet off the ground and hold your ankles parallel. Use your inner thigh muscles to hold your legs parallel to each other. (**SEE FIGURE 9-5**.)

ACTION Lower your chest toward the ground by bending your elbows, keeping your posture strong. Avoid dropping your head. (**SEE FIGURE 9-6**.) Straighten your arms and push your body up through your palms. Keep your shoulders relaxed. Maintain good alignment.

WEDDING WORKOUT POINTERS Inhale to prepare, exhale as you push up. Inhale, return to start. Place a towel under your palms to elevate them and reduce pressure on your wrists. Another option to reduce pressure on your wrists is to hold onto the dumbbells that rest on the floor. Avoid dropping your head. Your pushup should not resemble a nose dive. Avoid locking your elbows when you lift. Lower as far as possible.

VARIATIONS

(EASIER) Stand in front of a wall. Place your hands on the wall slightly wider than shoulder width apart. Bend elbows and lower body toward wall. Straighten arms as you push through hands.

(EASIER) On the floor, instead of working from a slanting board position, kneel on all fours. Lower your chest toward the floor by bending your elbows. Adjust the amount of the load by shifting more or less weight from your knees into your hands.

(HARDER) On the floor, instead of working from a slanting board position, extend your legs long and rest on the balls of your feet, so your body resembles a plank.

(HARDER) Place one end of the band under each of your hands and around your back. Push up against the increased resistance of the band. Lower with control.

Training Your Back

Training your back is essential to good health and to your wedding workout program. Strong back muscles, combined with trained abdominal muscles, prevent back pain and give you good posture. If you improve your posture, you will instantly look taller and as much as five pounds slimmer. Toning your back also provides muscle definition that can be shown off to its best advantage if you have an open back wedding dress.

Functionally, strong and healthy back muscles assist whenever you pull anything toward you. These muscles hold your torso erect and provide support when you sit so that you avoid pain from muscle fatigue. Your upper and mid-back muscles stabilize your scapula and support your shoulders. Strong back muscles are critical to injury prevention and help lower back pain—something you definitely want to avoid during your wedding and honeymoon.

Your back consists of several muscles. Your latissimus dorsi ("lats") is a large triangular shaped muscle that helps give the *V* shape to athletic backs. Your trapezius ("traps") is a large kite shaped muscle that spans the base of the neck, across your shoulders and down through your upper and mid-back. Across the upper back and in between your shoulder blades are the rhomboid muscles, which squeeze your shoulder blades together.

ONE-ARM ROW

Figures 9-7 and 9-8
One arm rows tone and strengthen your back, shoulders, and arms.

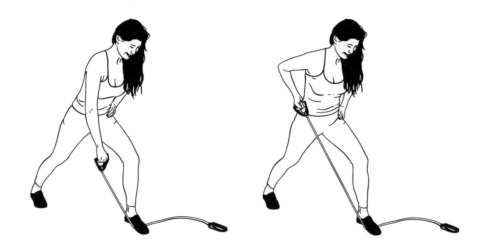

GET SET Stand in a generous split stance. Place one end of the band under your forward foot. Hold the other end of the band in your opposite hand with your palm facing downward and thumb pointing inward. Place the same hand as forward foot on mid-thigh for support. (**SEE FIGURE 9-7.**)

ACTION Slide your shoulders down and back. Bend your elbow as you pull your arm in toward your waist. Rotate your palm facing upward and thumb pointing outward. Slowly lower and return to start. (**SEE FIGURE 9-8.**)

WEDDING WORKOUT POINTERS Inhale to prepare, exhale to lift. Inhale, and return to start. Keep your abdominals pulled inward, shoulders down and relaxed. Avoid arching or sagging through your back.

VARIATIONS

(DUMBBELLS) While holding a dumbbell in your other hand, place the knee and hand of the same side of your body on a bench or chair like half of an "all fours" position. Maintain good alignment. Your hips and shoulders should be level. Allow the arm that is holding the dumbbell to hang directly below your shoulder without locking your elbow. Your palm should be facing inward. Keep your wrist joint flat. Bend your elbow and pull your arm up, while keeping your shoulder blade stabilized. Keep your elbow close to your body. Slowly lower.

LAT PULL DOWN

Figures 9-9 and 9-10

Lat pull downs tone and strengthen your back, arms, and shoulders. They also provide definition to your torso, creating a *V*-shape that enhances your waistline.

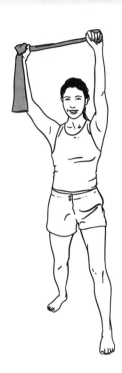
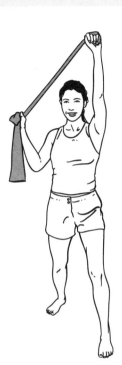

GET SET   Stand in a split stance with your feet hip-width apart and one foot slightly in front of the other. Hold one end of an exercise band or tubing in each hand in front of your body. Lift your arms overhead without hunching your shoulders with your palms facing forward. Pull in your abdominal muscles to support your lower back. (**SEE FIGURE 9-9**.)

ACTION   Pull your shoulders down and back. Keep your left arm elevated as you exhale and bend your right elbow in toward your waist. Feel the muscles under your arm and along the sides of your back contract. Keep your shoulders stable and your chest open. (**SEE FIGURE 9-10**.) Slowly return to start by raising your right arm.

WEDDING WORKOUT POINTERS   Inhale to prepare, exhale as you pull down. Inhale, return to start. Avoid arching your back or pulling the band or tubing by bouncing your torso back. Use your back muscles to pull the arm down. Keep your wrist joint flat.

RHOMBOID SQUEEZE

Figures 9-11 and 9-12
The rhomboid squeeze strengthens and tones your mid-upper back and arms. It improves posture by strengthening muscles that lift and open your chest.

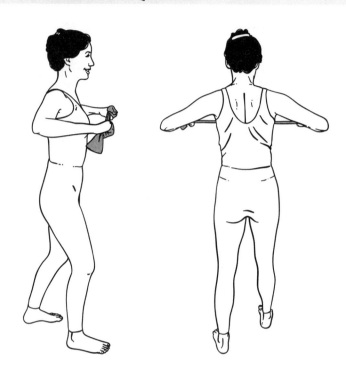

GET SET Stand in a split stance with your feet hip-width apart and one foot slightly in front of the other. Hold one end of an exercise band or tubing in each hand in front of your body. Reach forward and lengthen arms, with palms facing down, and arms horizontal and parallel to the ground. Pull in your abdominal muscles to support your lower back. (**SEE FIGURE 9-11.**)

ACTION Pull your shoulders down and back. Exhale as you bend your elbows and squeeze your shoulder blades together. Feel the muscles in between your shoulder blades contract. Keep your shoulders stable and your chest open. (**SEE FIGURE 9-12.**) Slowly return to start by straightening your arms and letting your shoulder blades spread wide.

WEDDING WORKOUT POINTERS Inhale to prepare, exhale as you squeeze. Inhale, return to start. Avoid arching your back, pulling the band, or hunching your shoulders. Keep your wrist joint flat.

DUMBBELL PULLOVER

Figures 9-13 and 9-14
The dumbbell pullover strengthens and tones your back and chest. It also provides a great stretch for the chest and rib cage.

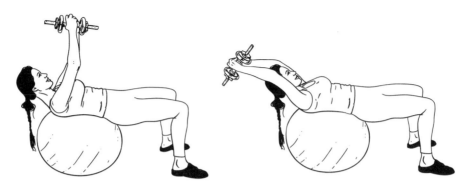

GET SET Lie on your back across a bench, chair, or stability ball with your knees bent and your feet on the ground, supporting the natural curve of your lower back. Tighten your buttocks and pull in your abdominal muscles to support your lower back. Keep your thighs parallel to the ground. Hold one dumbbell with both hands directly over your chest with your arms straight. Avoid locking your elbows. (**SEE FIGURE 9-13**.)

ACTION Pull your shoulders down and back. Inhale as you lower the weight in an arc past your head, keeping your rib cage in contact with the bench, chair, or ball by pulling in your abdominals. Go only as far as your shoulder flexibility permits. Avoid any pain or discomfort. Enjoy the stretch in your chest and rib cage. (**SEE FIGURE 9-14**.) Exhale as you lift the weight overhead in an arc until your hands are above your torso. Feel the muscles in your back working underneath your arms and along the sides of your torso. Inhale as you slowly return to start by lowering the weight in an arc past your head.

WEDDING WORKOUT POINTERS Avoid arching your back. Keep your wrist joint flat. Lying across a bench or chair is a more advanced position because your neck muscles need to be strong enough to comfortably support your head. Choose the stability ball option or wait until your neck muscles are stronger if you are unable to support your head comfortably.

VARIATIONS

To emphasize your chest muscles, bend your elbows more. To emphasize your back muscles, keep your arms as straight as possible.

Training Your Shoulders

Strengthening and toning your shoulder muscles prevents injuries and enhances your appearance in sleeveless and off-the-shoulder tops, which are common styles for wedding gowns. Another rewarding aspect of training your shoulder muscles is that they typically reveal visible results in a fairly short time, enabling you to enjoy "celebrity arms." While improving your appearance is a strong motivating factor, strong shoulders are very valuable in preventing injuries. This will come in handy on your honeymoon as you load and carry your suitcases.

Your shoulder muscles are known collectively as your deltoids or "delts" and include three muscles: your anterior, medial, and posterior deltoids, which means your front, center, and rear shoulder muscles. Your deltoids work together with the rotator cuff muscles to enable your shoulder to perform its broad variety of movements.

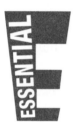

Women tend to fixate on the usual problem areas—like tummies, hips, and thighs. No surprise, then, that your back might be at the bottom of your shape-up list. Don't neglect it—wedding dresses often require elaborate undergarments that squeeze you through the torso. If you don't want a squashed-back visible beneath your gown, stick to these exercises!

The rotator cuff muscles include the supraspinatus, subcapularis, infraspinatus, and teres minor. If you strengthen these muscles, you will have stronger joints and more stable shoulders. This will prevent injury when you lift things or play sports.

OVERHEAD PRESS

Figures 9-15 and 9-16

The overhead press strengthens and tones the muscles of your shoulders, arms, and back. Defined shoulder muscles also enhance a V-shaped appearance and make your lower body appear more slender.

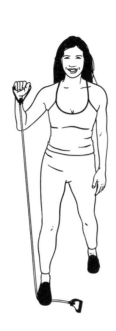 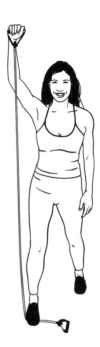

GET SET Stand in a split stance. Anchor one end of your band or tubing by standing on it with your right foot. Hold the other end of the band or tubing with your right hand. Tighten your abdominal muscles to support your lower back. (**SEE FIGURE 9-15**.)

ACTION Slide your shoulders down and back. Slowly press the band up with your other arm, palm facing forward, extending your arm fully without locking your elbow. Your arm will travel slightly forward. Keep your wrist joint flat. Maintain good alignment. Keep your abdominals tightened. (**SEE FIGURE 9-16**.)

WEDDING WORKOUT POINTERS Inhale to prepare, exhale to press up. Inhale, return to start. Tighten your abdominal muscles to stabilize your back.

VARIATIONS

(EASIER) Face your palms in, instead of forward.

(DUMBBELLS) Stand in a split stance. Hold a dumbbell in each hand. Bend your elbows, with your palms facing forward, and place your hands outside of your shoulders. It's like a "stick 'em up" position. Press weights up as high as you can go without locking your elbows. Lower to shoulder or slightly lower than shoulder height.

SIDE RAISE

Figures 9-17 and 9-18
The side raise strengthens and tones your shoulders and adds definition to the top central section, creating a wider shoulder line that eliminates the need for shoulder pads and slenderizes your lower body.

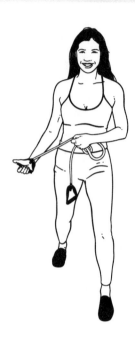
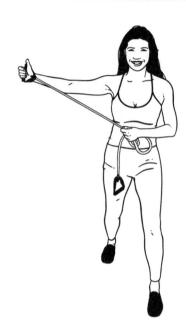

GET SET Stand in a split stance. Hold one end of an exercise band or tubing in each hand. Hold your left hand in the center front of your body with your right arm at your side, palm facing forward and thumb pointing up, as if you're a hitchhiker. (**SEE FIGURE 9-17.**)

ACTION Slide your shoulders down and back. Lift your right arm out to the side to approximately shoulder height. (**SEE FIGURE 9-18.**) Avoid locking your elbows. Keep your wrist joint flat. Lower slowly and with control.

WEDDING WORKOUT POINTERS Inhale to prepare, exhale to lift. Inhale to return to start. Lift arm directly to the side. Maintain good alignment. Keep abdominals pulled inward. Relax your shoulders. Keep your head level.

VARIATIONS

(EASIER) Perform while seated.

(DUMBBELLS) Stand in a split stance. Hold a dumbbell in each hand. Hang your arms at your sides with palms facing in. Lift your arms out to the side to approximately shoulder height. Avoid locking your elbows. Lower slowly and with control.

FORWARD RAISE

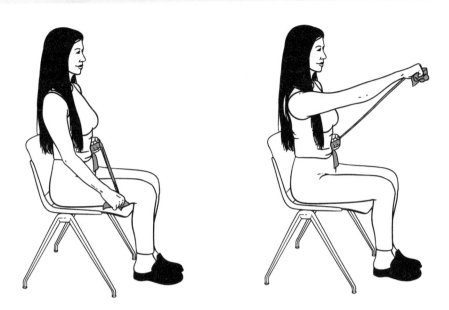

Figures 9-19 and 9-20

The forward raise strengthens and tones the front of your shoulders and chest.

GET SET Sit up straight in a stable, armless chair. Hold one end of an exercise band or tubing in each hand. Hold your left hand in the center front of your body with your right arm in front of your right thigh, palm facing backward. (**SEE FIGURE 9-19**.)

ACTION Slide your shoulders down and back. Raise your right arm forward, feeling the resistance of the band. Keep your wrist joint flat. Be sure to keep the opposite end stable. (**SEE FIGURE 9-20**.)

WEDDING WORKOUT POINTERS Inhale to prepare, exhale to lift. Inhale, return to start. Maintain good alignment. Keep your head level. Avoid rocking your body forward and back. Avoid arching your lower back.

VARIATIONS

(HARDER) Stand with legs parallel. It's more difficult to maintain good alignment.

(HARDER) Lie on your back on the floor.

(DUMBBELLS) Stand with feet hip-width apart. Use the split stance. Take one step back, bend both knees slightly, and balance your body weight between both legs and in the centers of your feet. Hold a dumbbell with a gentle grip in each hand. Slowly raise your arms in front of your body to shoulder height. Face your palms toward the ground. Keep your shoulders relaxed, abdominals pulled inward. Slowly lower weights back to start.

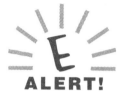

ALERT!

Remember to keep your back and abdominal muscles pulled in throughout all of your exercising. A strong core keeps your form steady and aligned. It also helps your body to work harder. You'll be rewarded in the end with an even stronger, flatter stomach for your wedding and honeymoon.

REAR SHOULDER FLY

Figures 9-21 and 9-22
The rear shoulder fly strengthens and tones the muscles in the back part of your shoulder and your mid-upper back.

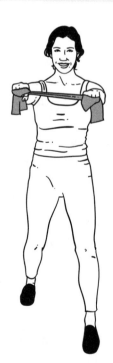
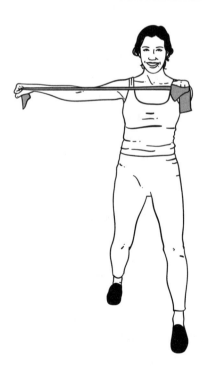

GET SET Stand in a split stance with your feet hip-width apart and one foot slightly in front of the other. Hold one end of an exercise band or tubing in each hand in front of your body. Reach forward and lengthen arms at shoulder height, with palms facing in, arms horizontal and parallel to the ground. Pull in your abdominal muscles to support your lower back. (**SEE FIGURE 9-21.**)

ACTION Slide your shoulders down and back. Pull your right arm back, feeling the muscles working in the back of your shoulder and in your mid-upper back. Keep your wrist joint flat and your shoulders and hips in alignment facing forward. Avoid twisting your torso. Be sure to keep the opposite end stable. (**SEE FIGURE 9-22.**)

WEDDING WORKOUT POINTERS Inhale to prepare, exhale to lift. Inhale to return. Move arm directly to the side. Maintain good alignment. Keep abdominals pulled inward to support your lower back. Relax your shoulders. Keep your head level.

VARIATIONS

(EASIER) Perform while seated.

(DUMBBELLS) Stand in a split stance with your upper body leaning forward at a forty-five–degree angle. Hold a dumbbell in each hand. Hang your arms straight down under your shoulders, palms facing in. Lift your arms out to the side just under shoulder height. Avoid locking your elbows. Lower slowly and with control.

Training Your Arms

Strengthening and toning your arms provides endurance when you carry things, prevents injuries of the wrist and elbow, and gives a healthy, firm look to your muscles. You'll appreciate this extra endurance when you are rushing around shopping for your wedding and need to be able to carry multiple bags on your forearm, or when you're working long hours on your computer, organizing your reception checklists. From an aesthetic point of view, firm, toned arms are attractive and give off an aura of healthful living. Because many wedding gowns are sleeveless, you can enjoy the results of your hard work on your wedding day as you proudly bare your arms and walk down the aisle.

The muscles in your forearm control your wrist and hand actions and the strength of your forearms determines your grip strength. Strengthening these muscles is not likely to win beauty points as you walk down the aisle, but you will score big in the functional fitness column. With everything else you have on your plate at the moment, the last thing you need to have to cope with is sore, aching wrists.

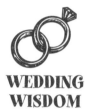

WEDDING WISDOM

When working your arms, be careful not to use jerky, uncontrolled motions. You'll need to move your arms comfortably to do many things during your wedding—like carry your bouquet, hug guests, and dance the night away with your groom. Those tasks won't be so easy if you pull muscles and can't raise your arms because of shoulder or back pain!

Like strengthening your shoulders, strengthening your forearms will not only help you to perform activities that use your hands but it will also help you do more exercises that require wrist stabilization. Strong wrists also help prevent injuries. Golfer's elbow or tennis elbow can be avoided by strengthening the forearm muscles, because strong muscles prevent excessive strain on joints. This is especially important if you're planning to take an active honeymoon or play recreational sports.

The main muscles in your arms are your biceps and triceps. Your biceps brachii actually works together with your brachialis. They are the primary muscles on the front of your upper arms. Your biceps is the bulging muscle in the upper arm that we most typically see in body building poses. The name biceps comes from the fact that the muscle has two heads. This means that it splits apart at the top of the muscle and attaches on the shoulder blade in two different locations. On the bottom of the muscle it attaches in one spot, on your forearm below your elbow joint.

The brachialis lies underneath your biceps. The brachialis is actually larger than your biceps, but because it is underneath, you can't really see it. It is also stronger than your biceps. One function of these muscles is to rotate your forearms. When you bend your elbow and turn your palms up or down, you are using your biceps and brachialis.

The triceps muscle is in the back of the upper arm located directly opposite your biceps and brachialis muscles. As you may have already guessed, the name triceps comes from the fact that the muscle has three heads. These heads all join in a shared tendon at the back of your elbow. The triceps heads include a lateral (outside of the arm) head, medial (inside of the arm) head, and long head.

The lateral head of the triceps runs from the back of the upper arm bone to the elbow. The medial head runs from the lower end of the arm bone to the elbow. The long head attaches on the shoulder blade, runs across the shoulder joint, and inserts at the elbow. For people who have a lot of muscle definition, you can actually see the contours from the different heads of the muscle.

If you're concerned about firming up the back of your arms, you want to be sure to include triceps exercises. You need to make an extra effort to exercise these muscles because most people do not challenge them a lot in their daily lives. One practical function of your triceps is to help you push yourself up and out of a chair with arms.

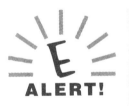

ALERT!

Your leg, thigh, and buttock muscles are probably the strongest in your body because you tend to use them more throughout the day. Daily activities don't generally require that you use your upper body a lot and, consequently, your arm and shoulder muscles are much smaller. Your weight level will be much lighter for these smaller, weaker muscles.

Always remember to train your triceps when you train your biceps. The synergistic work of the biceps and triceps is a perfect example of how our muscles work together. When your biceps contract, your elbow bends and your triceps muscles stretch. When you contract your triceps, your arm straightens out and your biceps muscles stretch. You can see how it is important to maintain balanced muscle development so one group of muscles does not overpower the other.

BICEPS CURL

Figures 9-23 and 9-24

The biceps curl strengthens and tones the muscles in the front of your upper arm.

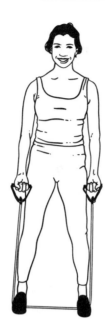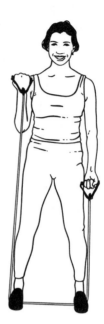

GET SET Stand on a band or tube with one foot. Hold the other end of band or tube with the hand on same side of the body. Stabilize your upper arm against your body. Begin with forearm parallel to floor, palm facing up. (**SEE FIGURE 9-23**.)

ACTION Lift your palm toward body against resistance. Keep wrist joint flat. Feel a strong contraction in your biceps muscle. Lower slowly. (**SEE FIGURE 9-24**.)

WEDDING WORKOUT POINTERS Inhale to prepare, exhale to lift. Inhale, return to start. Keep your upper arm stable. Do not rock your body or arch your back.

VARIATIONS

(EASIER) Perform exercise in a seated position.

(HARDER) Stand on band with both feet, one end in each hand. Anchor both upper arms against torso. Lift both arms at the same time. Lower slowly.

(DUMBBELLS) Stand in split stance. Hold a dumbbell in each hand with your palms facing away from your body. Stabilize your upper arms against your body. Maintain good alignment. Tighten your abdominals. Keep your wrist joints flat. Bend your elbows and raise the weights toward your chest. Lower slowly.

REVERSE BICEPS CURL

Figures 9-25 and 9-26

The reverse biceps curl strengthens and tones the muscles in the front of your upper arm and in your forearm.

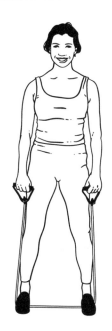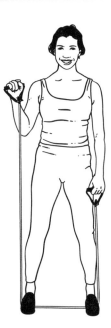

GET SET Stand on a band or tube with one foot. Hold other end of band or tube with hand on same side of the body. Stabilize upper arm against the body. Begin with forearm parallel to floor, palm facing down. (**SEE FIGURE 9-25.**)

ACTION Lift arm toward body against resistance so that palm faces forward. Keep wrist joint flat. Feel a strong contraction in your biceps muscle and in the muscle on the top of your forearm. Lower slowly. (**SEE FIGURE 9-26.**)

WEDDING WORKOUT POINTERS Inhale to prepare, exhale to lift. Inhale, return to start. Keep your upper arm stable. Do not rock your body or arch your back.

VARIATIONS

(EASIER) Perform exercise in a seated position.

(HARDER) Stand on band with both feet, one end in each hand. Anchor both upper arms against torso. Lift both arms at the same time. Lower slowly.

(DUMBBELLS) Stand in split stance. Hold a dumbbell in each hand with your palms facing backward. Stabilize your upper arms against your body. Maintain good alignment. Tighten your abdominals. Keep your wrist joints flat. Bend your elbows and raise the weights toward your chest so palms face forward. Lower slowly.

TRICEPS PUSHUP

Figure 9-27 and 9-28

The triceps pushup strengthens and tones the chest, shoulders, and arms. It firms and defines the muscles on the back of the upper arms.

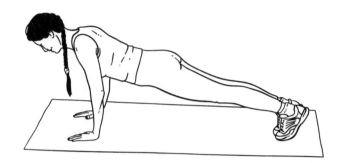

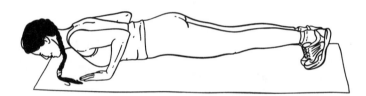

GET SET Kneel on all fours on the floor. Walk your hands forward until your hands are shoulder-width apart, your fingers point straight ahead, your elbows point toward your hips, and your torso resembles a slanted board. Tighten your abdominal muscles. Maintain good alignment. (**SEE FIGURE 9-27.**)

ACTION Bend your elbows toward your hips, keeping your arms close to your torso, and lower your upper body. Straighten your arms and push your body up through your palms, feeling the muscles working in the back of your upper arms. Keep your shoulders relaxed. Maintain good alignment. (**SEE FIGURE 9-28.**)

WEDDING WORKOUT POINTERS Inhale to prepare, exhale as you push up. Inhale, return to start. Place a towel under your palms to elevate palms and reduce pressure on your wrists. Avoid dropping your head. Avoid locking your elbows when you lift. Lower as low as possible.

VARIATIONS

(EASIER) Stand in front of a wall. Place hands on wall straight under shoulders, fingers pointing upward, and elbows pointing toward hips. Bend elbows, keeping arms close to your torso, and lower body toward wall. Straighten arms as you push through hands.

(EASIER) On floor, instead of working from a slanting board position, kneel on all fours in a tabletop position. Lower your chest toward the floor by bending your elbows. Adjust the amount of load by shifting more or less weight from your knees into your hands.

(HARDER) On floor, instead of working from a slanting board position on your knees, extend your legs straight and rest on the balls of your feet, so your body resembles a plank.

(HARDER) WITH BANDS OR TUBING) Assume same body position. Place one end of the band under each of your hands and around your back. Push up against the increased resistance of the band. Lower with control.

TRICEPS DIP

Figures 9-29 and 9-30

The triceps dip strengthens and tones your arms and shoulders. It also firms and defines the back of the upper arms.

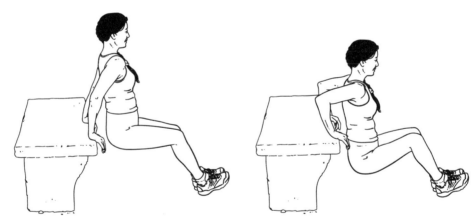

GET SET Sit on edge of chair or stable bench. Place hands on sides of chair seat. Slide your shoulder blades down and back. Walk feet out in front of your knees and rest on heels. Maintain good alignment. Slide your bottom off the chair seat. (**SEE FIGURE 9-29.**)

ACTION Make sure that your shoulders are stable. Slowly lower your hips as you bend your elbows to about ninety degrees. Push and lift hips up to starting position. (**SEE FIGURE 9-30.**)

WEDDING WORKOUT POINTERS Inhale to prepare, exhale and lower hips. Inhale, and return to start. Avoid allowing your shoulders to creep up to your ears. Tighten your abdominal muscles to stabilize lower back. If your wrists bother you, work on reverse biceps curls until your wrists become stronger.

VARIATIONS

(EASIER) Place your feet on floor closer to your body and bend your knees at a right angle. Perform exercise as described.

Chapter 10

Weight Training—Lower Body Exercises

The muscles of your lower body are absolutely essential to accomplish the simple tasks of everyday living such as walking, climbing stairs, getting up from chairs, and getting in and out of cars. As you prepare for your wedding and honeymoon, you're going to need plenty of energy and endurance. By doing these weight training exercises regularly, you'll sail through your wedding preparations and be ready for an active, fun-filled honeymoon. The fact that you'll look great in your shorts or swimsuit doesn't hurt either.

Training Your Hips and Buttocks

All of these exercises (in the hips and buttocks section and those that follow it) can be done at home or at the gym, whatever works best for your schedule. You can use dumbbells or bands and tubing and body weight to achieve the desired level of challenge. Whenever possible, each exercise presents multiple variations so that you can diversify your workouts over time and use whatever equipment that you have available. Strengthening and toning the muscles of your hips and buttocks provides you with more energy throughout the day, adds curves and definition to your lower body, and increases your metabolism. Because your buttock muscles are the largest muscles in your body, when these muscles are toned, you burn more calories even when you sleep. Strong buttock muscles also provide important support for your lower back, help prevent back pain, and improve your posture.

Building and keeping lower body strength ensures that you will enjoy independent living into your later years. Strong buttock muscles power your walk and help you get up out of chairs. Because many of us spend far too much of our time sitting due to the requirements of modern living, adding exercises to ensure the strength and endurance of these muscles is essential. You will immediately enjoy the benefits of your hard work when you discover that you have more energy and endurance to get through any physical activity.

The largest muscle group in your body is the glutei: maximus, medius, and minimus. These muscles are commonly referred to as the "glutes." As the name implies, your gluteus maximus is the largest. You use this muscle when you walk, run, or jump. Your gluteus maximus gives you the power in your stride. The gluteus medius is smaller and assists in more lateral movements such as side stepping. The more important function of the medial glute is in its role as a stabilizer for your hip joint because it keeps your pelvis level. The gluteus minimus is the smallest of the three muscles. When you rotate your leg outward from the hip, you use your gluteus minimus and your gluteus medius. These muscles are underneath what some people refer to as the "saddlebags" area.

SQUATS

Figures 10-1 and 10-2

Squats tone and strengthen your hips, buttocks, and thighs. They also firm and define the muscles that lift your bottom.

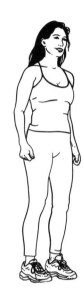
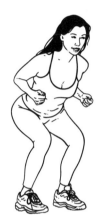

GET SET Stand with feet hip-width apart, pointing straight ahead. Pull in your abdominal muscles to support your lower back. (**SEE FIGURE 10-1.**)

ACTION Slide your shoulders down and back. Sit back as if you're going to sit in a chair. Do not bend your knees more than ninety degrees. To do this, make sure that your knees track over your feet, but do not go past your toes. Feel the muscles in the backs of your legs and in your hips and buttocks contracting. Keep your shoulders relaxed, abdominals pulled inward. (**SEE FIGURE 10-2.**)

WEDDING WORKOUT POINTERS Inhale as you sit back, exhale as you press up. Avoid arching your lower back by contracting your abdominals and pulling your lower ribs in toward your spine. Avoid arching your neck.

VARIATIONS

(**EASIER**) Use a chair or bench to spot you. Make sure that it is not too low. Sit back until you just feel your buttocks touch down. Push up through your heels.

(**EASIER**) Only lower half way to bench. Push up.

(**HARDER**) Perform the exercise while holding dumbbells in each hand.

(**HARDER**) Lift one knee up so thigh is parallel to the floor. Sit back into a one legged squat. Push up through heels. This is also a great balance challenge.

(**BANDS OR TUBING**) Stand on the center of a band or tubing while holding an end in each hand. Perform squat as described.

LUNGES

Figures 10-3 and 10-4
Lunges tone and strengthen your hips, buttocks, and thighs. This exercise provides firmness and definition to your thighs, too.

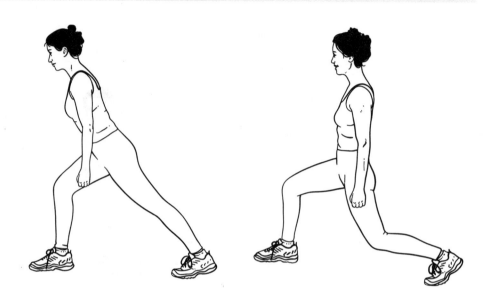

GET SET Stand with your feet hip-width apart. Take one generous step backward with your outside leg, keeping your legs hip-width apart in a large split stance. Stand on the full sole of your front foot and ball of your back foot. Pull in your abdominal muscles to support your lower back. (**SEE FIGURE 10-3**.)

ACTION Slide your shoulders down and back. Bend both knees to a ninety-degree angle as you lower your body toward the ground. Make sure that your front knee tracks over your foot and that it does not go beyond your toes. Your back knee will almost touch the floor. (**SEE FIGURE 10-4**.) Push up, feeling the weight in the heel of your front foot.

WEDDING WORKOUT POINTERS Inhale as you lower, exhale as you push up. Keep your abdominals pulled inward to support your lower back. Maintain good upright posture. If you need to lean forward, do so from the hips.

VARIATIONS

(EASIER) Use a wall or chair for support.

(HARDER) Hold a dumbbell in each hand.

(HARDER) Stand with feet hip-width apart to begin. Step forward with one leg into the lunge. Push off to return to start.

(HARDER) Step backward with one leg into lunge. Return to start. Can do either version with alternating legs.

(HARDER) Travel forward across the room as you lunge. Keep weight over heel of forward leg.

(BANDS OR TUBING) Step on the center of a band or tubing with your front foot. Hold an end in each hand. Perform lunge as described.

LEG PRESS BRIDGE

Figures 10-5 and 10-6

The leg press bridge strengthens and tones your buttocks and the backs of your thighs. It conditions your inner thighs as knee stabilizers and challenges your core muscles, which help you maintain good posture.

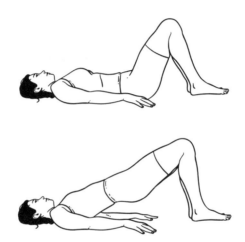

GET SET Lie on your back with good alignment, knees bent, with your feet comfortably close to your hips and hip-width apart. Place your arms straight at your sides with your palms down. **(SEE FIGURE 10-5.)**

ACTION Push through feet and lift your hips up off ground, squeezing your buttocks and muscles in the back of your thighs. Rest on your shoulders in a "bridge" position as you squeeze your buttocks at the top of the lift. Lower your hips to about one inch above the ground, keeping good alignment, to repeat the exercise. Do not lose your level pelvic position, hike one hip higher than the other, or arch your back. **(SEE FIGURE 10-6.)** Keep your shoulders relaxed.

WEDDING WORKOUT POINTERS Inhale to prepare, exhale as you push up. Inhale, return to start. Avoid arching your back or letting your legs open wide apart when you lift. Tighten your inner thighs to keep your legs straight.

VARIATIONS

(HARDER) While in the bridge position, lift your right leg up and place your ankle on your left thigh. Keep your weaker leg on the ground first. When you are finished, repeat the exercise with your stronger leg on the ground.

(HARDER) Assume same body position, except instead of resting your right ankle on your thigh, straighten your leg and reach up. Do exercise as described.

BENT-KNEE REAR LEG LIFT

Figures 10-7 and 10-8

The bent-knee rear leg lift strengthens and tones your buttocks and backs of thighs (your hamstrings). It challenges your core muscles to maintain good posture and adds firmness to the backs of your thighs.

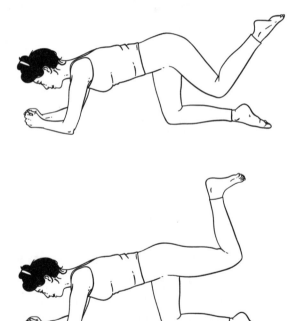

GET SET Kneel on all fours. Place elbows on floor under shoulders. Slide your shoulders down and back. Tighten abdominals to support your lower back. Maintain good alignment. Avoid dropping your head. (**SEE FIGURE 10-7**.)

ACTION Lift your left leg until your knee reaches hip height. Keep your hips and shoulders parallel to the ground. (**SEE FIGURE 10-8**.) Slowly lower.

WEDDING WORKOUT POINTERS Inhale to prepare, exhale as you raise your leg. Inhale as you return to start. Keep abdominals contracted, shoulders down and back, and neck lengthened.

VARIATIONS

(EASIER) Lie face down instead of on all fours. Place your forehead on the back of your hand. Avoid arching your back.

(HARDER) Add an ankle weight to the working leg.

(BANDS OR TUBING) Tie a band or tubing into a circle and place it around both feet at your instep. Do exercise as described.

Training Your Thighs

Training your thighs provides essential support to your knees and helps to prevent injuries. It also firms and defines the muscles of the upper leg, which is an aesthetic goal for many women. Strengthening the muscles of the back of your thighs combined with good nutritional habits can reduce the appearance of cellulite. Strong thighs also help you enjoy many active recreational pursuits such as hiking, tennis, skiing, and skating. Be sure to do these exercises to prepare for outdoor fun on your honeymoon.

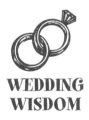

WEDDING WISDOM

If big, puffy wedding dresses loaded with layers of crinoline aren't your style, a straight-cut or A-line dress might be more your speed. These styles are striking and elegant, but you need the right shape to carry them off—they don't hide lower-body flaws like big skirts do. With these exercises, you'll look svelte and stunning in your stream-lined style.

Your quadriceps or quads are located in the front of your thighs. The quadriceps are actually four different muscles that work together. The quadriceps include the rectus femoris, vastus medialis, vastus lateralis, and vastus intermedius. You can see why people call them quads for short! The largest of your quads is the rectus femoris. The rectus femoris attaches at the hip joint as well as at the knee joint. The rectus femoris is part of your hip flexors because it lifts your upper leg when it contracts. Your quads allow you to extend your leg from the knee. One of the muscles in your quadricep group is also a hip flexor. Stretching your quads is important.

Your hamstrings are opposite to your quads. Your hamstring muscles are in the back of your thighs. The function of the hamstrings is to bend your knee and bring your heel toward your buttocks. Your hamstrings and glutes often work together to extend your leg behind you. Toned hamstrings and glutes improve your walking endurance for more energy every day.

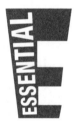

If feeling confident in a bikini is a goal for your honeymoon, pay attention to training your lower body. By paying as much attention to your lower body as you do to your midsection, you'll be able to ditch the sarong and show off strong quads and hamstrings, along with a toned bottom!

The muscles in your outer thighs are called hip abductors. When you contract your abductors, your leg moves away from your body. Your abductors along with the tensor fasciae latae muscle stabilize your hip and knee joints. For example, when you ride a bicycle, your abductors help keep your knee in line with your foot. Strong inner and outer thigh muscles also protect your knees and hips when you move from side-to-side. If you're a skier or tennis player, these muscles are particularly important to prevent knee injuries.

OUTER THIGH LEG LIFT

Figures 10-9 and 10-10

The outer thigh leg lift strengthens and tones the muscles in your hip and outer thighs and conditions the knee stabilizers. It also firms and tones the hip area.

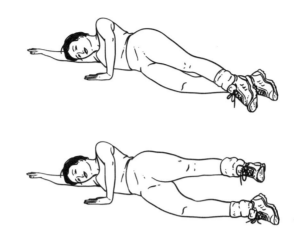

GET SET Lie on your side, placing your lower arm straight on your mat. Rest your head on your lower arm. Use your upper arm like a kickstand to support your body. Stack your hips perpendicular to the floor, pull in your abdominal muscles to support your lower back. Lengthen your top leg from the hip through the soles of your feet, with your leg parallel to the ground and your knees facing forward. (**SEE FIGURE 10-9.**)

ACTION Lift your top leg to hip height, keeping your pelvis stable. Avoid rolling forward or backward. (**SEE FIGURE 10-10.**) Slowly lower and return to start.

WEDDING WORKOUT POINTERS Inhale to prepare, exhale to lift. Inhale, return to start. Keep your abdominals pulled inward, shoulders down and relaxed. Avoid arching or sagging through your back.

VARIATIONS

Point your toes. Flex your feet.

(HARDER) Flex your foot and rotate your leg internally with your heel toward the ceiling. Lift.

(HARDER) Add ankle weights on your ankle or place on your outer thighs above your knee joint, if you have knee problems.

(BANDS OR TUBING) Tie your band in a circle or use a circular tube. Place around both thighs above the knee in side-lying position. Do movement as described.

INNER THIGH LEG LIFT

Figures 10-11 and 10-12

The inner thigh lift strengthens and tones your inner thighs, adding firmness and definition to your upper leg.

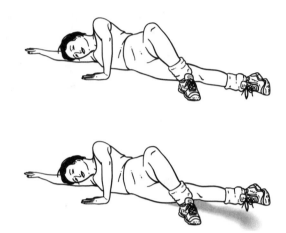

GET SET Lie on your side, placing your lower arm straight on your mat. Rest your head on your lower arm. Use your upper arm like a kickstand to support your body. Stack your hips perpendicular to the floor, pull in your abdominal muscles to support your lower back. Bend the knee of your top leg and place your foot on the ground with the knee of your bottom leg facing forward. (**SEE FIGURE 10-11**.)

ACTION Lift your lower leg up as high as possible without changing your alignment. Lengthen your leg through the bottom of your foot. Avoid tilting forward or backward. (**SEE FIGURE 10-12**.) Slowly return to start by lowering your leg.

WEDDING WORKOUT POINTERS Inhale to prepare, exhale as you lift lower leg. Inhale, return to start. Avoid arching your back and keep your shoulders down and back.

VARIATIONS

Instead of placing your top leg behind your lower leg, bend your knee and place in front of your body. You can rest your lower leg on a towel for support. Point your toes. Flex your feet.

(HARDER) Flex your foot and rotate your leg internally with your heel toward the ceiling. Lift.

(HARDER) Add ankle weights on your ankle or place them on your inner thighs above your knee joint, if you have knee problems.

(BANDS OR TUBING) Tie your band in a circle or use a circular tube. Keep top leg straight with knee of bottom leg slightly bent. Anchor under foot of top leg in side-lying position. Slip lower leg through loop. Perform movement as described.

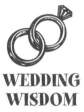

WEDDING WISDOM

You can hide your thighs under your dress, but there is still motivation for getting your legs toned. If you're having a garter toss, your legs will be the focus of the festivities for a few minutes. Get them in shape and you'll be excited and not skittish about it. You will also be ready to show them off on your honeymoon!

LEG CURL

Figures 10-13 and 10-14
The leg curl strengthens and tones the back of your thighs (your hamstrings).

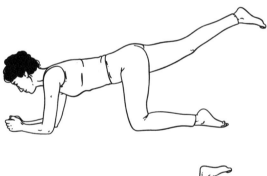

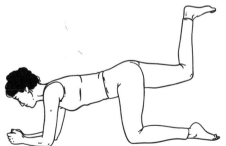

GET SET Kneel on all fours. Place elbows on floor under shoulders. Slide your shoulders down and back. Pull in your abdominal muscles to support your lower back. Avoid dropping your head. Extend right leg back with heel in line with buttocks. (**SEE FIGURE 10-13**.)

ACTION Lift right leg until your knee reaches hip height. Keep good alignment. Keep your hips and shoulders parallel to the ground. Bend your knee to raise heel toward buttocks. (**SEE FIGURE 10-14**.) Slowly return to start by straightening your right leg.

WEDDING WORKOUT POINTERS Inhale to prepare, exhale as you bend your knee. Inhale as you return to start. Keep abdominals contracted, shoulders down and back, and neck lengthened. Avoid arching your back.

VARIATIONS

(EASIER) Lie face down instead of on all fours. Place your forehead on the back of your hand. Avoid arching your back.

(HARDER) Add an ankle weight to the working leg.

(BANDS OR TUBING) Tie a band or tubing into a circle and place it around both feet at your instep. Do exercise as described.

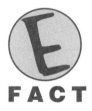

FACT

Women often complain about the hips, buttocks, and thighs as their most problematic areas. Not surprising, since women's bodies are built to carry fat in these places. These areas might seem like a tall order, but time spent targeting them will be well worth it. You'll gain confidence in your muscular curves instead of feeling self-conscious.

Training Your Lower Legs

Strengthening and toning your lower leg muscles improves your endurance for daily activities and most importantly, prevents injuries. It also enhances your ability to survive long stints in high-heeled shoes. Toned calves give shapely definition to the lower leg. If you're prone to building bigger muscles—a few women are—emphasize endurance training of your calves, rather than strength. Focus on higher reps and do not add additional weight.

Shins are not particularly glamorous or sexy, but strong shins prevent aches, pains, and injuries. If you've ever had shin splints, then you're intimately acquainted with these muscles.

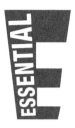

> You may think you exercise lower-body muscles enough in aerobic workouts, but you should also be training your lower body with weights. Although walking, running, hiking, biking, swimming, and other exercises put lower-body muscles to good use, it often takes more to really tone them. Some muscles in the lower body require targeted exercises to work them thoroughly and best shape them.

The muscles in the back of your lower leg make up your calves. The calf consists of two muscles, the soleus and the gastrocnemius. When you elevate onto the balls of your feet, you contract your calf muscles. Every time you lift your heels, you contract your calf muscles. That's why you may have felt muscle soreness in your lower legs after you went for long walk for the first time in awhile. Strengthening your calves will allow you to walk comfortably for longer periods of time.

Do not neglect your shin muscle, which is called the anterior tibialis. Your shins are in the front of your lower legs. If you've had shin splints or other lower leg problems in the past, it may be related to a muscle imbalance between your calves and shins. Like your biceps and triceps, your calves and shins work in relationship to each other. If you strengthen your calves, you should also strengthen your shins. Each time you pick up the ball of your foot, you contract your shins. Most people have overly tight calves and weak shins, so shin training should have even greater emphasis.

Stronger calves and shins increase mobility of your ankle joint. Flexible ankles play a crucial role in walking properly and maintaining your balance. Doing these exercises for the lower legs will improve your stability and reduce the risk of twisting your ankles or losing your balance. If you want to do more walking to improve your cardiovascular fitness and to lose weight, conditioning your calves and shins is essential so that you will have the endurance to survive long walks.

CALF RAISE

Figure 10-15

The calf raise strengthens and tones your calves. Defined calf muscles give shape to your lower leg.

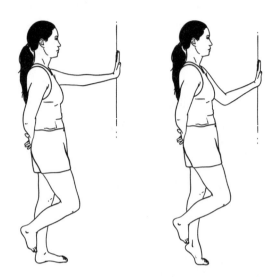

GET SET Stand behind a chair or facing a wall. Use your hands for support. Balance on the ball of your foot of the working leg. Wrap the other foot around the ankle of your working leg so that all of your weight is on one leg. (**SEE FIGURE 10-15**.)

ACTION Slide your shoulders down and back. Pull your abdominals in to support your lower back. Slowly push up onto the ball of your foot as high as you can lift. Maintain good alignment. Keep your abdominals tightened. Slowly lower without fully touching the floor.

WEDDING WORKOUT POINTERS Inhale to prepare, exhale as you push up. Inhale, return to start. Keep good posture throughout the movement.

VARIATIONS

Stand on a step so your foot is elevated from the floor. Place the ball of your foot on the step and let your heel hang off the edge. Slowly lower your heels before you begin, then push up as high as you can.

(EASIER) Do both legs together.

(HARDER) Do one leg at a time.

(HARDER) Hold a dumbbell in your hand to add more resistance than your body weight.

(HARDER) Use less and less hand support to challenge your balance. Progress to using only one fingertip or no support at all.

(BANDS OR TUBING) Sit on the ground with your legs straight ahead. Hold one end of a band or tubing in each hand. Place the center of the band around the sole of one foot. Extend your leg in front of you. Point and flex your foot. Feel the resistance as you point your foot. Maintain good seated posture.

TOE TAP

Figure 10-16

The toe tap strengthens and tones your shins.

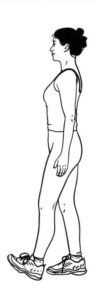

GET SET Stand comfortably.

ACTION Slide your shoulders down and back. Pull in your abdominals to support your lower back. Shift weight into your heels. Lift the ball of one foot as high as you can. (**SEE FIGURE 10-16**.)

WEDDING WORKOUT POINTERS Inhale to prepare, exhale to lift. Inhale, and return to start. Maintain good posture, with relaxed shoulders and a level head.

VARIATIONS

(EASIER) Perform while seated.

(HARDER) Lift balls of both feet at the same time.

(BANDS) Sit on a chair or the ground. Tie a band in a circle. Cross your ankles. Place the band over the top of the foot on the top leg. Keep the band in place by stepping on it with the foot of your lower leg. Point and flex your foot, feeling the shin muscle contract when you flex your foot.

Chapter 11

Core Training— Standing Tall and Confident

Core training helps you glide smoothly down the aisle, radiating confidence and grace. Core training is key to creating good posture, ease of movement, and balance and to avoiding aches and pains. By doing these core training exercises regularly, you'll be taller and slimmer in appearance and you'll feel like a million bucks. These results are well worth the minimal investment in time to fit these exercises into your busy schedule.

Why Core Training Is Important

Many people think that core training is simply another name for abdominal exercises, but this is incorrect. Core training is about training your body's foundation—the muscles that support good posture and efficient movement. Core training does not focus on a single muscle, but rather focuses on improving how the muscles at the center of your body work together to provide you with stability, balance, and control over your movement.

Core training focuses on building endurance in the muscles that support the spine, shoulders, and hips, and in improving the integration of how these muscles create stability. Earlier chapters focused on how to train some of these same muscles to improve specific muscular strength and endurance. This chapter focuses on how to train these muscles to work together to support the body as a singular unit. Well-trained core muscles improve every aspect of daily living, because whenever we are awake we benefit from movement control. In addition, you could say that core training even helps improve your slumber because you will avoid back pain and other aches that may disrupt restful sleep.

Modern living has taken many of the normal challenges to movement out of our lives such as walking on uneven surfaces and sitting without back support; therefore, it's necessary to incorporate core training into our daily routine to remind these muscles of the work that they need to do to provide stability. These exercises are the most important part of your program, because good alignment is essential to effective aerobic and weight training, as well as to every other aspect of your life. If you don't have time for anything else, always try to fit in some core training.

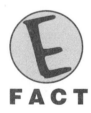

FACT

When you have good posture, your joints are properly aligned and you do not suffer excess strain in your neck, shoulders, back, hips or knees; you enjoy more efficient movement in all of your joints; you have better range of motion and flexibility from more balanced muscle development; and your internal organs function more efficiently.

Creating Good Posture and Stability

Core training creates good posture and stability in the body by targeting those muscles at the body's innermost layers. These muscles provide support to the spinal column, to the shoulders, and to the pelvis. The value of good posture goes far beyond looking attractive.

Improving Balance

Core training improves balance because it targets the deep muscles of your abdominals and your lower back, which are responsible for your body's sensitivity to where you are in space. For example, if you lose your footing, these muscles at the innermost layers of your spine react quickly to readjust your weight distribution and restore your balance. Improving the tone of these muscles goes a long way to prevent accidents. Investing in training your core helps ensure that you won't trip down the aisle as you stroll gracefully down to meet your fiancé!

Preventing Aches, Pains, and Injuries

Most adults suffer from back pain at some point in their life. It's the leading cause of disability from work in the United States. Because you're under considerable stress with all the preparatory tasks for your wedding and honeymoon, you want to be sure that you avoid back pain. Core training targets the muscles of the back, abdominals, and pelvic floor to ensure good posture. This training helps you to stand and sit properly, avoid tension in the neck and shoulder area, and to lift and carry things without straining your back or shoulders.

Improving Your Sex Life

Studies show that becoming more fit in general improves your sex life. Core training, specifically, tones up your pelvic floor and deep abdominals, restores spinal flexibility, and improves control over your pelvis, which all together adds up to more enjoyment from sex. Not only will you have more endurance, you'll also enjoy more sensitivity. This is a great benefit for any married couple.

Core Training Guidelines

Core training exercises differ from other weight training exercises by focusing exclusively on building endurance, rather than on creating strength and endurance. The reason for this is that your deep stabilizer muscles are made up of almost 100 percent slow twitch fibers that are designed to be working at all times. Unlike other mover muscles that are geared toward short bursts of work, your stabilizer muscles need to be working all of your waking hours. In addition, because core training works on improving movement efficiency, attention to form is critical.

The following are general guidelines for your core exercises:

- **Train for endurance:** Do between twelve to twenty reps depending on the specific exercise. Certain exercises such as the plank are held for thirty seconds or more. Work up to two to three sets if time permits.
- **Emphasize control and perfect form:** Focus on perfect form with every rep. Stop doing the exercise when you are unable to maintain form, regardless of the number of reps.
- **Exercise daily:** Incorporate a few core exercises on a daily basis to remind you to use the muscles that keep good posture at all times.
- **Combine with stretching:** Stretch at the same time that you do your core exercises to improve flexibility and to enhance balanced muscle development.

Keep these guidelines in mind as you do your core stabilization exercises.

Training Your Core

Core muscles include a variety of back, abdominal, hip, and pelvic floor muscles that work together to stabilize the body. Some of these muscles, such as the deepest layer of the abdominals, play only a stabilizing role. Other muscles, such as the outer layer muscles of the abdominals, play an important part in assisting larger movements such as bending forward. What is different about training core muscles is that the focus is on how these muscles work together, rather than improving individual strength of any particular muscle.

Your trunk stabilizer muscles include the transversus abdominus, the deepest layer of abdominal muscles, the internal obliques, which lie above the transversus, the multifidus, and quadratus lumborum, deep muscles of the lower back, and the erector spinae, which support the entire length of the spine.

When you take a deep breath and pull your belly button toward your spine as you exhale, you are activating your transversus. This muscle is large and covers the area under your ribs, around your abdomen, and above your pelvis. When the transversus contracts, it pulls in the belly in a three-dimensional fashion, like nature's girdle to support the lower back. This muscle's primary function is to support your organs and your spine. When you cough or sneeze, you can feel your transversus contract.

The erector spinae and multifidus muscles attach to your spine. These muscles are located along the spine in the upper, mid- and lower back. Your erector spinae run from your neck all the way to your hips on both sides of the spine. They also branch off and attach at your ribs and spine in the mid- and upper back. These muscles enable you to bend backwards, sideways, and to rotate your torso. Because we don't do a lot of backward bends during the day, these muscles mostly work as stabilizers to support our lower backs as we sit, walk, or run. These stabilizers are working in all of the exercises that require you to maintain neutral spinal alignment. Back extension exercises are the best way to challenge the erector spinae muscles to work as primary movers.

The shoulder stabilizers include the trapezius and rhomboids, discussed in Chapter 9, and other smaller muscles that support the shoulder joint. The pelvic stabilizers include muscles of the hips and buttocks, the gluteus medius, minimus, and tensor fascia latae, discussed in Chapter 10, and the pelvic floor muscles. Some researchers also believe that the diaphragm, which is a breathing muscle, also provides stability to the pelvis.

The pelvic floor muscles span the bottom of the pelvis. These muscles support our internal organs. Most important, these muscles maintain bladder control and contribute to sexual health in both men and women.

To exercise and strengthen your pelvic floor muscles, combine the following with each of your core body exercises. As you do your abdominal and lower back exercises, when you exhale, contract your pelvic floor muscles as you pull your deep abdominal muscles inward. When you inhale, release.

PELVIC TILT

Figures 11-1 and 11-2

The pelvic tilt tones your abdominals, lower back, and buttocks. It also improves spinal flexibility in the lower back.

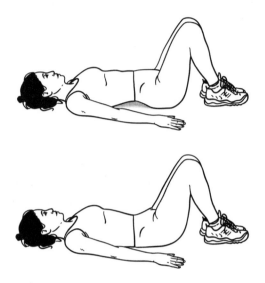

GET SET Lie on the ground with your knees bent at a ninety-degree angle, with your feet flat. Start with good alignment keeping the natural curve in your lower back. Place your arms at your sides. (**SEE FIGURE 11-1**.)

ACTION Slide your shoulders down and back. Contract your abdominals by pulling inward. Notice that your lower back tilts back and flattens. Keep your shoulders relaxed. (**SEE FIGURE 11-2**) Relax your abdominals and return to start.

WEDDING WORKOUT POINTERS Inhale to prepare, exhale as you tilt your pelvis. Inhale, return to start. Lift your pelvic floor as you exhale and contract your deep abdominals. Feel the stretch in your lower back. Notice if you are squeezing your buttocks to tilt your pelvis. Focus on using more abdominal muscles to move your hips, instead of your buttocks.

VARIATIONS

Pelvic Clock—Imagine that your lower back and hips create a clock face. Behind your navel is twelve o'clock and the tip of your tailbone is six o'clock. Roll your pelvis around the clock face in both directions. Feel abdominals working.

HEEL DIP OR DYING BUG

Figure 11-3

The heel dip, also called the dying bug, strengthens and tones the abdominal area. It conditions muscles that stabilize and support the lower back.

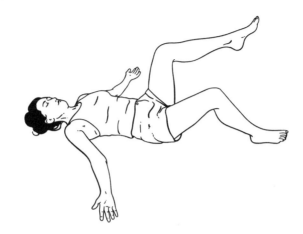

GET SET Lie on your back with good alignment, knees bent, and feet comfortably close to your hips and hip-width apart. Place your arms at your sides with your palms down. Lift your right knee above your hip with your knees bent at ninety-degrees, keeping your pelvis level and the natural curve in your lower back.

ACTION Lower your right leg, moving only from the hip joint, until your right heel touches the ground. (**SEE FIGURE 11-3**.) Lift your right leg back to start position. Repeat with left leg. Continue slowly alternating foot taps for thirty seconds.

WEDDING WORKOUT POINTERS Inhale as you lift your leg, exhale as you lower it. Avoid arching your back or "popping" your rib cage off the ground. Keep shoulders relaxed.

VARIATIONS

(HARDER) Lift one leg as you lower the other, rather than waiting for the leg to return to start position.

(HARDER) Increase the angle of your knee joint to more than ninety degrees up to a straight leg as long as you can keep your pelvis level and rib cage grounded.

ALL FOURS SPINAL STABILIZATION

Figure 11-4

All fours spinal stabilization tones your core stabilizer muscles. It improves posture.

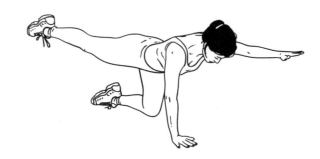

GET SET Kneel on all fours, hands under shoulders, and knees under hips. Maintain good alignment.

ACTION Contract your abdominals. Extend arm and opposite leg straight out in front and behind. Maintain good alignment, especially through the neck. Hold for six to ten seconds. (**SEE FIGURE 11-4.**) Slowly lower.

WEDDING WORKOUT POINTERS Inhale to prepare, exhale as you lift your arm and leg. Keep your navel pulled toward your spine throughout the exercise. Lift your pelvic floor as you contract deep abdominals. Avoid dropping your head. Avoid arching your back.

VARIATIONS

(EASIER) Do one arm at a time. Do one leg at a time. Concentrate on maintaining good alignment.

(HARDER) Repeat three to five reps on same side before doing the opposite side without placing your knee and hand fully on the ground.

PLANK

Figure 11-5

The plank strengthens and tones your core stabilizers. It improves posture.

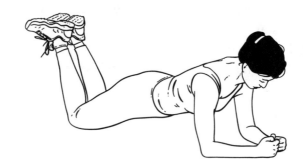

GET SET Kneel on all fours. Place your forearms on the floor, palms down, and elbows under shoulders. Walk knees out behind hips.

ACTION Contract your abdominals. Push up onto your knees into a plank position. Maintain good alignment. Hold up to thirty seconds. (**SEE FIGURE 11-5.**)

WEDDING WORKOUT POINTERS Inhale, to prepare, exhale, lift pelvic floor up as you contract your deep abdominals. Breathe naturally as you hold position. Inhale, return to start. Avoid arching your neck or lower back.

VARIATIONS

(HARDER) Lengthen your legs and roll up onto toes, similar to a full pushup position.

BRIDGING

Figure 11-6

Bridging tones the muscles in your abdominal area and buttocks. It improves spinal mobility.

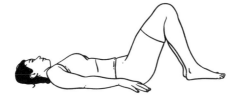 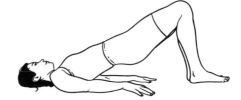

GET SET Lie on your back with good alignment, knees bent, and with your feet comfortably close to your hips and hip-width apart. Lay your arms straight at your sides with your palms down. (**SEE FIGURE 11-6.**)

ACTION Tilt your pelvis and continue the tilting motion, lifting your spine off ground, one vertebra at a time, stopping when you reach your shoulders. Slowly lower your spine one vertebra at a time and return to start. Repeat five to six times.

WEDDING WORKOUT POINTERS Inhale to prepare, exhale as you lift and lower your spine. Keep your jaw, neck, and shoulders relaxed.

BACK EXTENSION

Figure 11-7

The back extension strengthens and tones the lower back and the muscles that support the spine.

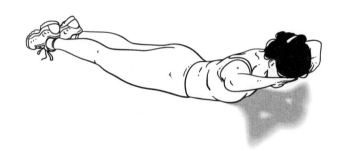

GET SET   Lie facedown on your stomach. Place a towel under your hips to support your lower back. Slide your shoulder blades down. Place your hands under your forehead.

ACTION   Contract your abdominals. Lift your chest off the floor as you slide your shoulder blades down. (**SEE FIGURE 11-7.**) Lower to start.

WEDDING WORKOUT POINTERS   Inhale to prepare, exhale, lift your pelvic floor, and contract your deep abdominals. Inhale, lift your torso. Exhale, return to start. Avoid arching your neck. Do not do this exercise if you experience any pain.

VARIATIONS

(EASIER) Lengthen arms along sides. Do exercise as described.

(HARDER) Add a rotation at the top of the lift. Rotate shoulder back, return to center, and roll down. Repeat on the other side.

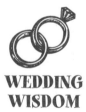

WEDDING WISDOM

It might be tempting to try to manage all of your wedding tasks on your own, but there will come a point when you're juggling too many balls in the air, and your stress levels will shoot up. Don't go it alone, and don't be afraid to delegate—as long as you do it nicely, of course!

SIDE PLANK

Figure 11-8

The side plank strengthens and tones the abdominal area (including the abs along your sides, called obliques) and the trunk and shoulder stabilizers.

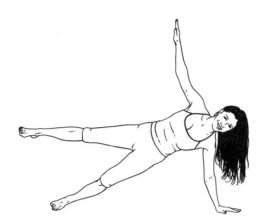

GET SET Recline on your right side with your right elbow bent 90 degrees and placed directly under your shoulder. Place your top arm, palm down, in front of your body. Your legs should be straight, with the foot of your top leg, in front of the foot of the lower leg.

ACTION Push down through your elbow, lifting your hips off the ground, and sweep your top arm straight up into a side plank position. Keep your back and neck long. Tighten abdominal muscles, keeping your buttocks tight to stabilize pelvis and lift lower hip upward. Do not relax muscles and collapse into shoulder. Keep your chest and back open wide. Lift your top leg until it is parallel to the floor. Look up at the elevated arm. (**SEE FIGURE 11-8**.) Work up to a thirty-second hold.

WEDDING WORKOUT POINTERS Inhale to prepare, exhale as you push up. Breathe normally as you hold.

VARIATIONS

(EASIER) Bend knee of bottom leg and lift up onto elbow and knee.

REVERSE PLANK

Figures 11-9 and 11-10
The reverse plank strengthens and tones your trunk and shoulder stabilizer muscles. It also tones your triceps.

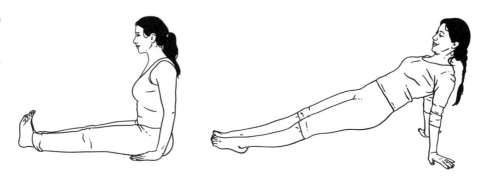

GET SET Sit with your hands palms down outside your hips, fingers facing any direction that is comfortable, with your legs straight, heels on ground. (**SEE FIGURE 11-9**.)

ACTION Slide your shoulders down and back. Pull in your abdominals to support your lower back. Push your heels into ground as you lift hips up into a plank position. Squeeze buttocks and hamstrings to lift hips. Straighten arms, avoid locking elbows, stabilize shoulders, look straight ahead or relax your neck and hang your head down and back. (**SEE FIGURE 11-10**.)Hold for up to thirty seconds.

WEDDING WORKOUT POINTERS Inhale to prepare, exhale to lift. Breathe naturally as you hold. Choose neck position that is most comfortable.

VARIATIONS

(EASIER) Start with your knees bent and feet flat. Push up so that your torso resembles a tabletop.

Training Your Abdominals

Your abdominal muscles support good posture as stabilizers and enable you to bend and twist at the waist as primary mover muscles. Abdominal training gives your belly a flatter appearance by providing muscular support, but it does not spot reduce excess fat that may lie over the muscles. When training abdominals for stabilization purposes, follow core training guidelines. When training abdominals as movers, follow training guidelines for building a combination of strength and endurance or endurance alone, depending on your individual goals. Most women prefer to build smooth, flat abdominals. To avoid creating bulky, sculpted abs, keep the rep range high with between fifteen and twenty-four reps for each exercise and avoid adding extra weight.

Your abdominal muscles are located in front of the torso and consist of four muscles. The muscle that people see in photos of "six-pack" abs is the rectus abdominis. It has tendonous sheaths within the muscle that create a lined appearance. It attaches under your breastbone and runs down to your pubic bone. Your rectus abdominis allows your torso to bend forward. Whether you can see your rectus abdominis underneath your skin depends on a number of factors. The single most important factor is genetics.

Your genetics determine the extent of muscularity that you can build and determine the location of your body fat deposits. Some people naturally store more fat under the skin on top of the rectus abdominus muscle, which makes it difficult to see the muscle development. Others tend to store more body fat in other areas of the body.

A second factor that determines whether you can see muscle definition under your skin is your body composition. Your body composition is the relative amount of lean body mass and fat mass that make up your body. If you have a low percentage of body fat, your muscles will be more visible under the skin. Similarly, if you have a high body fat percentage, you will not be able to see much muscle definition under the skin. The third factor is your training.

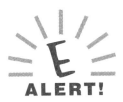
ALERT!

The most common example of muscle imbalance is focusing on training abdominals. In order to strengthen the mid-section, it's equally important to train the muscles in back as well as in front. If you only train abdominals, you can set yourself up for injury, postural misalignment, and potential back pain.

Underneath your rectus abdominus, you have two layers of oblique muscles. One layer runs at an angle down and in toward the center and another runs up and in toward the center. The function of your obliques is to bend and twist your torso. These muscles also assist in defining your waist. The movement that most commonly leads to lower back injury is bending and twisting. This is when your spine is most vulnerable. Strong oblique muscles protect your spine in this movement and help prevent back injuries.

CRUNCH

Figure 11-11

The crunch strengthens and tones your abdominal area and defines the muscles at the center of the torso.

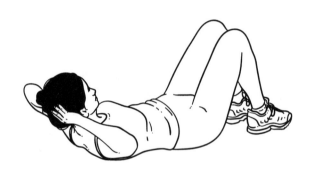

GET SET Lie on the ground with your knees bent, feet flat. Maintain good spinal alignment with the natural curve in your lower back. Place your fingertips behind your head with your elbows out wide.

ACTION Slide your shoulders down and back. Lift your head and upper back as you bring your lower ribs toward your pelvis. Contract your abdominal muscles. Lower slowly. (**SEE FIGURE 11-11**.)

WEDDING WORKOUT POINTERS Inhale to prepare, exhale as you lift up. Inhale, return to start. Avoid pulling on your head and straining your neck. Lift pelvic floor as you exhale and contract your deep abdominals.

VARIATIONS

(EASIER) Place your arms at your sides and lift upward as you slide your hands toward your feet.

(EASIER) Hold on to your thighs to assist you in lifting your torso forward.

(HARDER) Extend your arms behind you, past your ears. Lift and lower as described. If you feel discomfort in lower back, try bringing your feet closer to your hips.

(HARDER) Hold a dumbbell across your chest under folded arms.

REVERSE CRUNCH

Figures 11-12 and 11-13

The reverse crunch strengthens and tones the abdominal area and targets the lower abdominal area in particular.

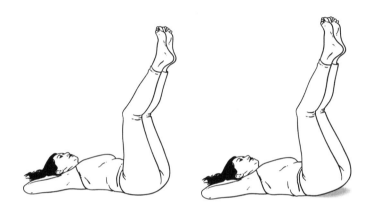

GET SET   Lie on your back. Bend knees with thighs perpendicular to ground and shins parallel. Place hands at your side, on either side of your head, or across your chest. **(SEE FIGURE 11-12.)**

ACTION   Slide your shoulders down and back. Contract your abdominals and curl your tailbone up and in-between your legs as you lift your hips upward. Lower slowly. **(SEE FIGURE 11-13.)**

WEDDING WORKOUT POINTERS   Relax your chest and shoulders. Avoid bouncing your hips up. Smoothly lift and lower. Relax your face, jaw, and neck. Lift pelvic floor as you exhale and contract your deep abdominals.

VARIATIONS

(HARDER) Do on an incline slant board with your head higher than your hips. Place your hands above your head and gently hold on to handle. Gradually increase the incline.

(BANDS OR TUBING) Start in bent knee position. Hold one end of the band in each hand. Place band across the top of your mid-thighs, above your knees. As you lift hips up, feel resistance to the movement as you work against the band. Lower slowly.

OBLIQUE CRUNCH

Figure 11-14

The oblique crunch strengthens and tones the rotator muscles of the trunk. It narrows and defines your waist.

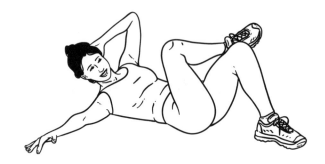

GET SET Lie on your back with your knees bent at a ninety-degree angle, feet flat on the ground. Place one hand behind your head with your elbow out. Extend opposite arm out to side of body, palm down.

ACTION Contract abs. Lift shoulder toward opposite knee, keep elbow out. Rotate the torso. Return to start. (**SEE FIGURE 11-14.**)

WEDDING WORKOUT POINTERS Inhale to prepare, exhale rotate and lift. Inhale, return to start. Concentrate on lifting your shoulder toward the knee and not on bending the elbow. Keep your abdominal muscles pulled inward as you rotate. Lift pelvic floor as you exhale and contract your deep abdominals.

VARIATIONS

(EASIER) If you have discomfort in your lower back, bring feet closer to hips.

(EASIER) Extend your arms long. Imagine you are peeling your shoulder up off the floor as you reach with both arms toward the outside of your legs. Alternate sides, or do reps on one side, then the other.

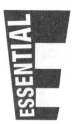

Strong muscles give you energy to get up and go. When you get stronger, you're also likely to become more active. As your strength increases, all of your daily activities will seem easier. This increased activity boosts your metabolism and increases the number of calories that you burn.

BENT KNEE SIDE CRUNCH

Figure 11-15

The bent knee side crunch strengthens and tones the trunk rotator muscles. It narrows and defines the waist.

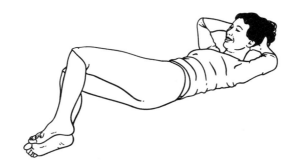

GET SET Lie on your back with your knees bent and feet flat. Lower both knees to one side, keeping your legs stacked together. Place fingertips behind your head. Place thumbs at base of hairline.

ACTION Curl upward, drawing your ribs toward your hips and squeezing your waist on one side. (**SEE FIGURE 11-15**.) Lower slowly.

WEDDING WORKOUT POINTERS Inhale to prepare, exhale to lift. Inhale, return to start. Avoid pulling on your neck.

VARIATIONS

(DUMBBELLS) Hold a light dumbbell behind your head.

BICYCLE

Figure 11-16

The bicycle strengthens and tones the abdominal area, particularly the waist. It defines and narrows the waist.

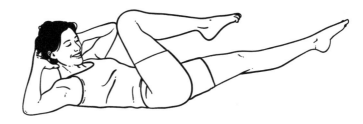

GET SET Lie on your back. Bend knees with thighs perpendicular to ground and shins parallel. Place fingertips behind head, elbows out wide, and shoulders down and back. Rotate upper body to the right, lifting left shoulder toward the right knee as you draw right knee in and extend left leg. Keep pelvis anchored. (**SEE FIGURE 11-16**.)

ACTION Switch legs, rotating your upper body to the left, lifting right shoulder toward the left knee as you draw left knee in and extend right leg. Keep rotating and switching knees toward chest.

WEDDING WORKOUT POINTERS Inhale as you lift alternating knees to your chest left and right, exhale as you lift alternating knees to chest left and right. This equals one repetition. Keep pelvis anchored at all times, rotating through the waist, not turning your hips.

VARIATIONS

(EASIER) If you cannot keep your pelvis still, do oblique crunches.

Chapter 12

Stretching—Being Limber and Serene

Being flexible makes you feel good, physically and mentally, reduces your risk of injuries, aches, and pains, and contributes to good posture and graceful movement—all important benefits for you as you approach your wedding and honeymoon. Stretching regularly is key to maintaining your flexibility. Flexibility is joint specific, so you need to include stretches for the major muscle groups of your body. In the busy months before your wedding, enjoy your stretching as a relaxing time out to refresh both your mind and your body.

Stretching for a Better Body and Mind

Stretching lengthens your muscles, increases fullness of movement at your joints, releases muscular tension, and encourages physical and mental relaxation. When you're limber, you can move freely, bend over easily, and smoothly turn your head. When your muscles are not flexible, you feel tight and stiff, and everyday movements can be painful or difficult.

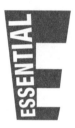

If you have a short torso, stretch as much as possible. Wedding dresses are usually heavily constructed through the waist. Any elongating you can do for your torso just might help you to achieve a better, smoother fit without any buckling or puckering at the waist. You just might save time and money on alterations, too!

A modern lifestyle that requires long hours of sitting or repetitive motions contributes to muscular tension and stiffness. Most people lose flexibility as they age, but this is not inevitable. If you start stretching regularly now, you can maintain your youthful limberness over the years of your life.

Stretching provides many benefits, including the following:

- Increases full and free movement
- Improves balance and proprioception, which is awareness of where your body is in space
- Encourages balanced muscle development which increases joint stability
- Reduces risk of injury and muscle soreness
- Improves posture
- Prevents lower back pain
- Alleviates muscle cramps
- Improves joint health by lubricating joints when moved through a full range of motion
- Improves athletic performance

- Enhances weight training by preventing feelings of tightness or stiffness
- Relieves muscle pain and tension
- Increases feelings of well-being
- Increases mind-body awareness so you're more able to detect tension
- Enhances feelings of relaxation

Stretching can deliver these results in minutes at a time, making it well worth your attention.

Factors That Affect Flexibility

Stretching benefits all body types, and it isn't necessary that you be able to bend yourself into a pretzel to enjoy these rewards. As you've probably noticed, some people are simply more flexible than others. Flexibility has a strong genetic component, and is affected by age and gender. Women are typically more flexible than men. If you're not a naturally flexible person, however, don't give up.

Factors that you can control that affect flexibility include your level of physical activity and muscle temperature. Your muscles are likely to be more healthy when you lead an active lifestyle. Regular activity ensures frequent movement, good circulation, and good muscle tone. Staying active helps you to improve your flexibility.

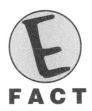

FACT

Proprioception has big implications for your wedding. If you consider yourself a klutz or just can't seem to get around without tripping and bumping into things, pay close attention here. A better sense of where your body is spatially will help you as you walk down the aisle, position yourself for photos, enter your reception, and dance with your groom.

The second factor over which you can exert control is muscle temperature. In general, a warm muscle experiences a better and more lasting response to stretching than a cold muscle. For best results, include stretches after every training session regardless of whether it is an aerobic or weight training workout.

For weight training sessions, mix stretches in between sets to target muscles that you've just worked. You can also stretch at the end of your cardio workout as part of your cool down. Either way prevents muscle soreness and enhances conditioning benefits. Stretching at the end of a workout will increase your feeling of relaxation.

Don't wait until your workouts, however, to enjoy a stretch. While you won't gain as much flexibility from simply stretching throughout your day, you will keep your joints healthy and release muscle tension. It's a good idea to enjoy a stretch break every hour for a few minutes. Take every opportunity that you can to fit in stretches during your day—while waiting in lines, sitting at stop lights, or walking across the office. The more often you stretch, the better you will feel.

Stretching Techniques and Tips

Stretching has a low risk of injury and stretching regularly can reduce the likelihood of injuries. The key to preventing injury is to use safe techniques. The wedding workout focuses on static stretching because it's the safest method of stretching, is easy to do, and is effective. For static stretching, move gently and deliberately through your natural range of motion. Ease off if you feel any joint strain. You should feel the stretch in the muscles, not the joints. Hold each stretch to a point of moderate tension—with no pain—in the target muscle. Hold each stretch fifteen to thirty seconds.

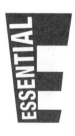

Maintaining your mental flexibility is a must when it comes to coping. The more you learn to let things roll off your back, the more you'll ultimately enjoy the planning process and your big day. No wedding goes off without at least a few little hitches. And often, these things are what make weddings memorable!

Your breathing pattern is also important to enhancing your stretch. As you inhale, increase the feeling of lengthening the muscle; when you exhale, hold or deepen the stretch as you feel muscular tension releasing. Try to lengthen your breathing rhythm. For example, inhale for up to four to five seconds and exhale for up to five or six seconds or longer. This rate of breathing—a ten-second breath cycle—stimulates the relaxation response. The result is that your heart rate and blood pressure become lower and the levels of stress hormones flowing in your blood stream decline. To stimulate the relaxation response, hold each stretch for a minimum of three deep breath cycles.

Avoid forced or rapid movements. Do not bounce when you stretch. Repeated bouncing, especially of cold muscles, increases the risk of tearing your muscles. Choose slow, static holds to get the best results. As you stretch, release tension from other parts of your body, such as your shoulders, jaw, chest, and neck.

Props can be useful to help stretch tight muscles and to increase comfort. Use a stretch strap or towel to help you stretch tight muscles in your upper or lower body. For upper body stretches, you can hold a strap behind your back with one end in each hand to stretch the chest and shoulders. For lower body stretches, you can place the center of a strap underneath the ball of your foot and hold one end in each hand. When using a strap, be sure to avoid trying to force any stretch. Still work within your natural range of motion and hold all stretches to the point of moderate tension.

Upper Body Stretching Exercises

Stretching the upper body is particularly important to prevent rounded shoulders and a collapsed chest and to release tension from the neck, shoulders, and upper back. Frequent sitting as part of a modern lifestyle causes most people to slouch and to hold tension in their necks and shoulders. To counteract these tendencies, be sure to do your weight training exercises for the back, shoulders, and chest, and include stretches to open up the chest and shoulders and release tension from the neck, shoulders, and upper back.

SEATED CHEST AND SHOULDER STRETCH

Figure 12-1

The seated chest and shoulder stretch releases muscular tightness in the chest and front of shoulders.

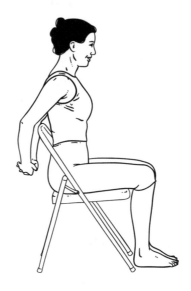

GET SET   Sit comfortably in your chair, shoulders relaxed, arms at your sides. Clasp hands together behind your back. Pull in abdominals to support your lower back.

ACTION   Squeeze shoulder blades together and gently lift hands to open up your chest and shoulders. (**SEE FIGURE 12-1.**)

WEDDING WORKOUT POINTERS   Inhale as you expand your chest, exhale as you squeeze your shoulder blades together and deepen the stretch. Avoid arching your lower back or straining your shoulders.

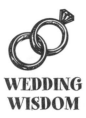

WEDDING WISDOM

Flexibility is not only about fitness—it's a state of mind. Just as you train your muscles to relax and loosen up through stretching, remain flexible with wedding planning. Maybe you'll need to choose different flowers if your first choice isn't in season. Or maybe you need to change your reception time because of availability. Unexpected things always pop up—be willing to adapt.

SEATED TRICEPS AND BACK STRETCH

Figure 12-2

The seated triceps and back stretch releases muscular tightness in the back, shoulder and upper arm.

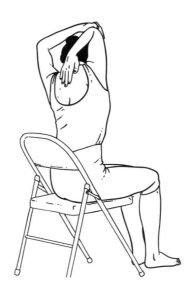

GET SET Sit comfortably in your chair. Lift your right elbow upward as you slide the palm of your right hand behind your neck. Place left hand on your right elbow.

ACTION Rotate internally at your waist and lift up and over with your elbow, lower your chin toward your chest, and press the back of your arm gently with your left hand. (**SEE FIGURE 12-2.**) Keep your abdominals tight to support your lower back. Feel the stretch in the back of your arm, in your upper back, and along the side of your torso.

WEDDING WORKOUT POINTERS   Inhale as you lengthen, exhale as you rotate and deepen the stretch. Keep abdominals pulled in to support lower back. Concentrate on lifting and lengthening, rather than collapsing into the torso.

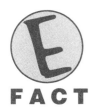

FACT

Most people spend too much time stressing out at their desks or racing around when they're on the go. This all adds up to plenty of pent up muscle tension. The more attuned you are to detecting this tension, the faster you'll be able to take a deep breath and prevent it or stretch to relieve achiness.

CAT STRETCH

Figure 12-3

The cat stretch releases muscular tension from your upper, middle, and lower back and in the neck and shoulders.

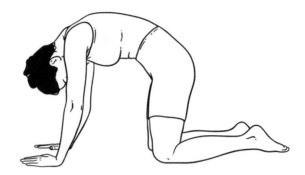

GET SET Kneel on all fours with hands under shoulders and knees under hips. Lengthen through neck and torso.

ACTION Round your spine by tucking in your tailbone. Spread shoulder blades wide and relax your neck by letting your head hang. (**SEE FIGURE 12-3.**)

WEDDING WORKOUT POINTERS Inhale as you lengthen and exhale as you round your spine. Flow through the motion without holding the straight or rounded positions, feeling flexibility in your spine. Hold the rounded position and gently turn your head side to side for an additional stretch in the neck and shoulders.

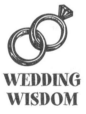

WEDDING WISDOM

Planning to wear high heels to your wedding? Do plenty of calf stretches. Also bring a cute pair of flats for the reception. Wear your heels through the ceremony and pictures, and then change shoes for the reception. Wedding dresses are so long, no one will even notice the switch!

Lower Body Stretching Exercises

Stretching out your lower body can prevent lower back pain and greatly enhance freedom of movement in the hip joints. In addition to contributing to a slouching posture, sitting for long hours at a time leads to inflexibility in the hips, tightness in the lower back, the buttocks, hamstrings, and calves.

Wearing high heels regularly also contributes to tight calves. If you like wearing high heels, try to vary your heel heights. For example, one day wear high heels, the next day wear flats, and on the third day, wear a medium-high heel. Be sure to stretch out your calves at the end of the day and do toe taps to keep your shins strong.

STANDING CALF STRETCH

Figure 12-4

The standing calf stretch stretches the back of the lower leg and improves ankle flexibility.

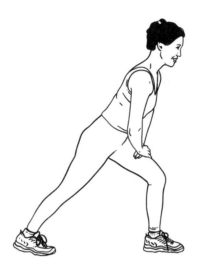

GET SET   Stand in a long split stance with feet hip-width apart. Place hands on mid-thigh of forward leg for support. Avoid putting any pressure on your knee joint.

ACTION   Push heel of back leg into ground as you straighten leg and lengthen torso. Feel the stretch in the back of your lower leg. (**SEE FIGURE 12-4**.) Keep abdominals tight to support lower back. Increase the stretch by sliding your heel further back.

WEDDING WORKOUT POINTERS   Slide back foot only as far back as you can keep your heel touching the ground. Keep your back foot parallel to your front foot and lengthen behind your knee. Avoid pointing toes outward. Shorten stance if necessary to keep foot pointing forward.

LYING HAMSTRING STRETCH

Figure 12-5

The lying hamstring stretch releases muscular tightness in the back of the upper leg. If the foot is flexed, it also stretches the back of the lower leg.

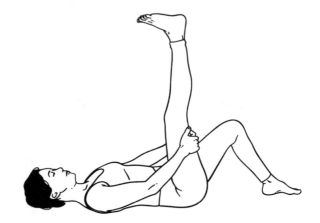

GET SET Lie on your back with both knees bent and feet flat on ground. Draw right knee toward chest with hands behind upper thigh. Straighten leg without locking knee joint and lengthen leg upward through heel.

ACTION Draw top of thigh toward chest. Feel stretch in the back of your upper leg. (**SEE FIGURE 12-5.**)

WEDDING WORKOUT POINTERS Exhale as you deepen the stretch. Flex foot to increase stretch in back of lower leg.

SIDE-LYING HIP FLEXORS AND QUADRICEPS STRETCH

Figure 12-6

The side-lying hip flexors and quadriceps stretch stretches the front of the hip and the thigh.

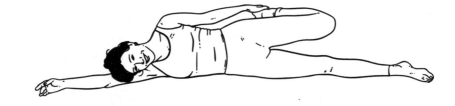

GET SET Lie on your side with your bottom arm extended as a support for your head. Place a strap or your hand around your foot or ankle. Tighten your abdominal muscles and keep your pelvis in a neutral position to provide support for your lower back and to prevent arching.

ACTION Bend the knee of your top leg as you draw your heel toward the buttocks. Feel the stretch in the front of your hip and thigh. (**SEE FIGURE 12-6**.)

WEDDING WORKOUT POINTERS Keep both knees parallel to each other. Be sure to feel the stretch in the front of the hip and thigh. If you feel any strain in your knee, ease up on the stretch until you feel it only in the muscle.

DEEP BUTTOCKS STRETCH

Figure 12-7

The deep buttocks stretch stretches the deep muscles of the buttocks and hips and can help prevent sciatica (shooting pains in the back of the legs).

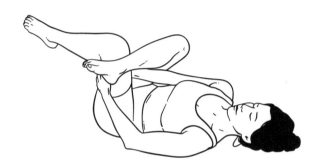

GET SET Lie on your back with knees bent. Pull your right knee toward your chest and place your right ankle on top of your left thigh. Your leg configuration resembles a number 4. Place both hands around back of your left thigh.

ACTION Pull your left thigh toward chest. Feel stretch deep in the buttocks and hips. (**SEE FIGURE 12-7**.)

WEDDING WORKOUT POINTERS Because this muscle area tends to be tight, ease gently into your stretch. This stretch can prevent or relieve sciatica due to pressure of tight muscles against the sciatic nerve.

Total Body Stretching Exercises

Stretching your entire body is a great tension reliever that can help you relax your muscles and feel refreshed. The more you do these stretches, the more sensitive you will be to tension in your body. Over time, you'll learn how to keep your muscles more relaxed. This gives a great result during the hectic days of wedding planning.

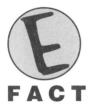

FACT

Sciatica is something worth avoiding. The intense, shooting pains it sends through hips and down legs can make it tough to get around, bend, and do simple tasks. Especially if you plan an active honeymoon and want to maintain an active lifestyle, stretch whenever you can to prevent it.

In addition to releasing tension, total body stretches elongate the torso for a slenderizing effect. Do these exercises consistently to avoid collapsing into and shortening your waist. Take time to do these full body stretches on a daily basis in your bed before you get up or at the end of the day.

FULL LENGTH TORSO CRESCENT STRETCH

Figures 12-8 and 12-9
The full length torso stretch stretches the abdominal area, back, legs, and arms.

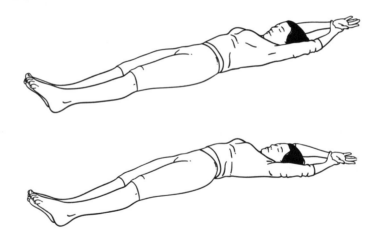

GET SET Lie on your back with your legs lengthened and your arms resting overhead. Clasp your right wrist with your left hand. (**SEE FIGURE 12-8.**)

ACTION Slide your arms and legs to the left, creating a crescent shape. Feel the stretch along the entire right side of your torso. (**SEE FIGURE 12-9.**)

WEDDING WORKOUT POINTERS This is a feel good stretch that lengthens the entire body, especially the waist. Emphasize lengthening the lowest rib away from your hip bone.

Chapter 13

Mind-Body Training— Yoga and Pilates

Your mind and body are profoundly intertwined. Certain types of exercises, like yoga, tai chi, qigong, and Pilates, tap more deeply into this relationship if practiced with focused attention. When movement becomes more meditative, it brings deeper benefits that go beyond merely toning or working your body. You find your source of inner calm, heighten your body awareness, and touch your deepest essence or spirit—all of which are valuable to you as your wedding approaches.

What Is Mindful Movement?

Mind-body styles of training, or mindful movement practices, offer a holistic way to train your entire body as an integrated unit, as well as focus your mind and improve your relationship with your mind, body, and spirit. Most styles of mind-body training come from ancient Eastern disciplines that were practiced as both a form of self-care and as a means to attain spiritual enlightenment. These movement methods are characterized by the following:

- Attention to breath
- A sense of knowing where the body is in space
- Concentration on the body and its movement
- Focus on proper form and technique
- Present state awareness
- Discovery of inner peace and the body's wisdom
- Connection with the energy of life

Incorporating mindful training into your program gives you the benefits of these tried and true systems of wellness.

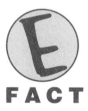

FACT

More than eighteen million Americans practice yoga and/or tai chi, and more than 10 million Americans practice Pilates. Tai chi is the most enduring and popular form of group exercise practiced by millions worldwide.

For purposes of the wedding workout, this chapter includes both yoga and Pilates exercises that you can use in your program. For more complete instruction, however, it's best that you find a reputable studio in your neighborhood and sign up for a weekly class. The exercises provided here give you a small taste of what each of these disciplines can do for you. If you find that you enjoy them or are interested in learning more, check out the resources in Appendix D to help you find local instructors. Be sure to start with a class that is for beginners to avoid frustration and possible injury.

Yoga and Its Benefits

The physical practice of yoga, known as *hatha yoga*, emerged in India more than 5,000 years ago as an approach to living developed from the spiritual practices of Vedic people. The term *yoga* comes from Sanskrit and means "union." According to Vedic principles, yoga is a union of body with mind and mind with spirit. In the Vedic system, achieving unity or inner harmony leads to self-realization. Self-realization ultimately leads to self-transcendence or unity with the One or Universal Spirit, which is considered the highest level of spiritual evolution. To dedicate one's self to practicing yoga, therefore, is to dedicate one's self to pursuing enlightenment. People who follow a yogic lifestyle seek to include yogic principles in daily living.

While yoga's philosophy embraces principles of spirituality, yoga itself is not a religion. Accordingly, the practice of hatha yoga should not interfere with any particular belief system and can be practiced by followers of any faith or by people who are spiritual, but not religious.

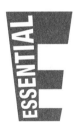

People of all ages, sizes, and levels of ability can benefit from the practice of yoga. Modifications exist for every posture. Find a well-qualified instructor who knows how to tailor the exercises to meet your needs and does not expect you to do anything that is uncomfortable. Be sure to communicate openly with your instructor about your individual circumstances.

The practice of hatha yoga consists of a series of poses, known as *asanas,* that you hold anywhere from a few seconds to several minutes. The moves require a blend of strength, flexibility, and body awareness and are intended to promote union of body, mind, and spirit and to prepare the body for the discipline of meditation and other spiritual yoga practices.

The consistent practice of yoga provides numerous physical and mental health benefits according to a large and growing body of research. Scientists, interested in the link between mind and body, or how thoughts and feelings can affect physiology, conduct research in the field of mind-body medicine. Because yoga is a leading form of mind-body exercise—a movement discipline that combines mindful techniques with physical movements—it has been the focus of much medical scientific interest.

Studies of yoga report the following benefits:

- Improved physical health
- Better sleep
- Effective stress and anger management
- Reduced responsiveness to stress hormones
- Decreased pain and pain sensitization
- Greater sense of well-being
- An overall improved mental outlook

Most hatha yoga styles include the same basic poses but differ in terms of how quickly you move, how long you hold each pose, how much breathing is emphasized, and how much of a spiritual aspect is involved. In the Indian tradition, all physical yoga is hatha yoga. In contrast, in America, different styles of hatha yoga have been given new names such as power, flow, or hot yoga. Other styles are named after the individual people who spread the exercise in America. For example, Iyengar yoga, named after B.K.S. Iyengar, is the most widely practiced style of hatha yoga in America and offers modifications for beginners.

Sample Yoga Exercises

To give you a sampling of what practicing yoga is like, several asanas, or postures, are provided here. The first set of moves comprises the sun salutation and is frequently used in Yoga classes as a warm up before doing more vigorous postures. Traditionally, it's practiced first thing in the morning, facing toward the sun. Before you do the sun salutation, it's a good idea to prepare your body with some gentle stretches. This can consist of doing each of the postures first slowly and separately before linking them together as a dynamic sequence.

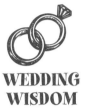

WEDDING WISDOM

Yoga teaches you not to collapse in your shoulders, which is especially important if you have an off the shoulder or sleeved gown. Any gapping you have where your dress fits around the shoulders won't be attractive—and it could be quite noticeable in pictures. Keep those shoulders straight, back, and relaxed—and don't hunch!

The sun salutation is one of the most popular yoga sequences. Once you memorize it, it's an excellent sequence to practice to keep your body limber and allow you to move with ease. Doing the sun salutation on a regular basis provides the following benefits:

- Warms up all major muscle groups
- Warms up and lubricates the joints
- Stretches and strengthens your spine and its supporting muscles
- Stretches and strengthens your arms and legs
- Regulates and coordinates breath with movement
- Connects body, mind, and breath
- Stimulates cardiovascular system
- Increases circulation
- Tones the diaphragm and other breathing muscles
- Eliminates stiffness
- Restores feelings of calm alertness or wakefulness

Flow smoothly from one posture to the next. Repeat for three to six cycles.

1. **Mountain Posture:** Inhale as you stand upright with good posture, feet hip-width apart. Arms relaxed at your sides. (**SEE FIGURE 13-1.**)
2. **Exhale:** As you breathe out, place the palms of your hands together at the center of your chest, with your thumbs touching your breastbone. (**SEE FIGURE 13-2.**)
3. **Backward Bend:** Inhale as you sweep your arms overhead with palms facing in. Look up and lift your chest upward. Keep your shoulders relaxed. (**SEE FIGURE 13-3.**)
4. **Forward Bend:** Exhale as you slowly bend forward, reaching your arms forward and down, palms facing front and then resting on the ground. If you can't touch the ground, bend your knees until you can. Align your fingertips with your toes. Bring your nose to your knees. (**SEE FIGURE 13-4.**) If your back is not strong enough to support your extended arms, roll down, leading with your hand, and keep your arms at your sides.

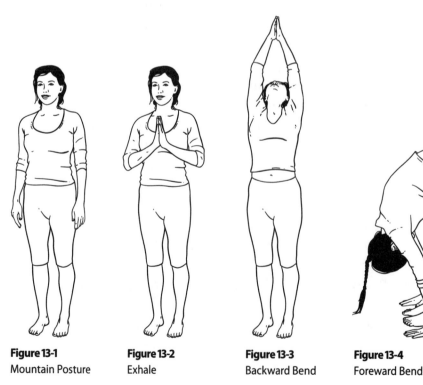

Figure 13-1
Mountain Posture

Figure 13-2
Exhale

Figure 13-3
Backward Bend

Figure 13-4
Foreward Bend

5. **Lunge:** Inhale, as you step backward with your left foot, lowering your left knee to the ground into a lunge position. Your right foot remains in between your hands, fingers aligned with the toes. Your right knee is directly above your right ankle. (**SEE FIGURE 13-5**.) If your right knee angle is less than 90 degrees, use your left hand to lift your right ankle and place your foot forward.

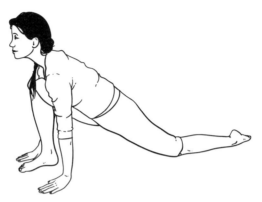

Figure 13-5
Lunge

6. **Plank:** Retain your breath as you step backward with your left foot onto the ball of your foot, lowering your hips into a plank position. (**SEE FIGURE 13-6**.) If it's too difficult to hold the plank position on the balls of your feet, lower your knees to the ground into a modified plank position.

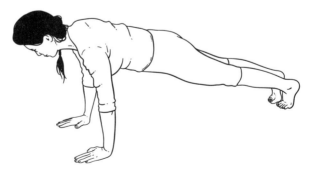

Figure 13-6
Plank

7. **Eight-Point Posture:** Exhale, as you lower your knees, chest, nose, and fore-head to the ground. Your buttocks remain up in the air. (**SEE FIGURE 13-7**).

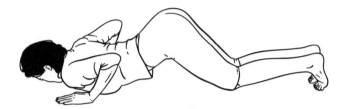

Figure 13-7
Eight-Point Posture

8. **Cobra:** Inhale, as you lower your hips, slide your shoulders down, and look up as you lift your chest upward into a cobra position. (**SEE FIGURE 13-8**.) Your legs and hips remain on the ground. Avoid hunching your shoulders.

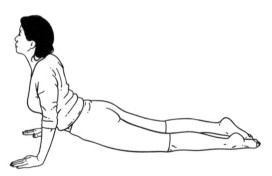

Figure 13-8
Cobra

9. **Downward-Facing Dog:** Exhale, lift your hips up, and draw your abdominals inward into an inverted-*V* position. Spread your fingers wide and press your palms into the ground. Lower your heels to the ground. (**SEE FIGURE 13-9.**) Do not force your heels to the ground if your calves are too tight. Modify by bending your knees slightly as you continue to lift the bottom of your pelvis, your sitz bones, upward.

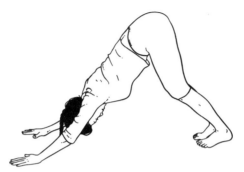

Figure 13-9
Downward-Facing Dog

10. **Lunge:** Inhale, as you step forward with your right foot into a lunge position, lowering your left knee to the ground into a lunge position. Your right foot is in between your hands, fingers aligned with the toes. Your right knee is directly above your right ankle. (**SEE FIGURE 13-10.**) If your right knee angle is less than ninety degrees, use your left hand to lift your right ankle and place your foot forward.

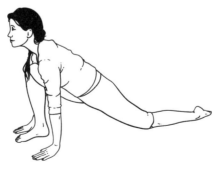

Figure 13-10
Lunge

11. **Forward Bend:** Exhale, as you bring your left foot forward next to your right foot, lifting your hips into the air with your nose to your knees in a forward bend position. (**SEE FIGURE 13-11.**)

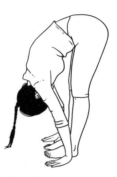

Figure 13-11
Forward Bend

12. **Backward Bend:** Inhale, as you sweep both arms upward into an upright position, with palms facing in, lifting your chest upward, and looking up. (**SEE FIGURE 13-12.**) If your back is not strong enough to support your extended arms, roll up slowly, keeping your arms at your sides or providing even more support for your back by walking your hands up your legs.

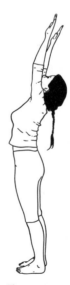

Figure 13-12
Backward Bend

13. **Mountain Posture:** Exhale, as you lower your arms to your sides and return to an upright position.

14. Repeat the complete sequence, except lead with the left leg as you step back into a lunge and again with the left leg as you step forward into a lunge. After you finish leading with each leg, you have completed one round of the Sun Salutation.

CHILD POSTURE

Figure 13-13

The child posture releases lower back tension and gently stretches the spine and neck.

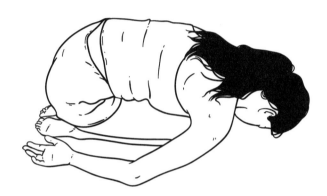

GET SET Kneel on all fours with hands under shoulders and knees under hips. Lengthen through neck and torso.

ACTION Lower your hips toward your heels as far as is comfortable for your knees. Lower your forehead to the floor and place your arms at your sides, palms facing up. (**SEE FIGURE 13-13.**)

WEDDING WORKOUT POINTERS Exhale as you lower your hips toward the heels. Inhale, breathe deeply, and feel a sense of expansion in your rib cage and lower back. Yield to gravity as you let your shoulder blades melt wide across your back. Soften the muscles around your eyes, jaw, and throat. Allow tension to drain away from your body with each exhalation.

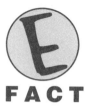

FACT

All forms of exercise boost self esteem and confidence through mastery of activity and body strengthening. However, exercises that tap into the mind-body connection maximize these benefits. Connecting with your true self will make you the most confident you can be as you learn to be comfortable allowing your authentic self to shine through in all you do.

EXTENDED CHILD POSTURE

Figure 13-14

The extended child posture stretches the neck, chest, shoulders, and lower back. It also gently elongates the spine.

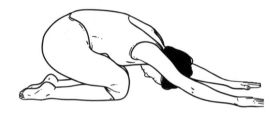

GET SET Kneel on all fours with hands under shoulders and knees under hips. Lengthen through neck and torso.

ACTION Lower your hips toward your heels as far as is comfortable for your knees. Walk your hands out straightening your arms for the longest possible stretch along your back. (**SEE FIGURE 13-14**).

WEDDING WORKOUT POINTERS Exhale as you lower your hips toward the heels. Inhale, breathe deeply, and feel a stretch in your upper back, chest and shoulders. Continue to breathe deeply, releasing lower back tension.

KNEE HUG

Figure 13-15

The knee hug release lower back tension and stretches the hips and buttocks

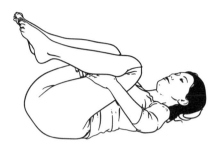

GET SET Lie on your back with your knees bent, feet on the ground, and arms at your sides. Place arms around the backs of your thighs.

ACTION Draw both knees toward your chest. Relax your lower back into the ground. (**SEE FIGURE 13-15.**)

WEDDING WORKOUT POINTERS Exhale as you draw your knees closer to your chest. For a lower back massage, gently circle legs, feeling the massage in your lower back, hips, and at the base of your spine. If necessary to avoid arching your neck, place a small pillow or rolled towel under your head.

VARIATIONS

To get more of a stretch through your inner thighs, draw your knees outward toward your shoulders.

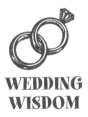

WEDDING WISDOM

Focusing your attention and remaining in the present are great goals. It's easy to get swept up in wedding tasks and lose sight of enjoying the process. Resist the urge to dwell on what's already done—the past— and don't angst over what you've yet to tackle—the future. Enjoy every step along the way as you're in the moment.

SINGLE-KNEE HUG

Figure 13-16

The single-knee hug releases lower back tension and stretches the hip and buttocks. It also stretches the hip flexors at the top of the thighs.

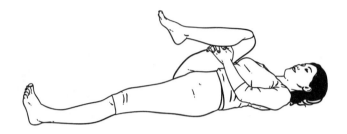

GET SET Lie on your back with your knees bent, feet on the ground, and arms at your sides. Place both arms around the back of one thigh.

ACTION Draw one knee toward your chest. Slide your other leg out straight. Keeping your leg on the ground, flex your foot, and press down gently through the heel. Relax your lower back into the ground. (**SEE FIGURE 13-16.**) Release stretch and place foot on ground with knee bent. Repeat with the other leg.

WEDDING WORKOUT POINTERS Exhale as you draw your knee closer to your chest. Soften your chest, shoulders, throat, and jaw, allowing any excess tension to drain away. If necessary to avoid arching your neck, place a small pillow or rolled towel under your head. If your back is particularly tight, the single knee variation is more comfortable than the knee hug with both legs simultaneously.

VARIATIONS

(SEATED) Sit comfortably in your chair and place arms around the back of one thigh. As you exhale, draw your knee toward your chest, keeping your other foot on the ground. Breathe deeply and release tension in your lower back and buttocks.

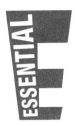

This is where your reality check comes in. Forget about which colors your bridesmaids paint their nails or—heaven forbid—what will happen if a few clouds float your way on your wedding day. Focusing on the mind-body-spirit connection will help you to see the real meaning of things—like the love you and your groom share and the commitment you're making.

Pilates and Its Benefits

Pilates is a form of exercise developed by Joseph Pilates and introduced in the United States in the 1920s. Pilates was a former boxer and self-defense trainer with extensive physical training. The Pilates method of exercise blends influences from yoga, Chinese acrobatics, gymnastics, and boxing. The key difference between yoga postures and Pilates mat exercises is that Pilates mat classes involve a series of specialized calisthenic exercises, so you're focusing on targeted muscles rather than the flow of energy in your body. Pilates also created a number of innovative training machines including the Reformer and the Trapeze Table, among others. The Reformer resembles a cot with springs, straps, and a sliding carriage, and was based on devices he created when he worked in a hospital. The Trapeze Table looks like a four-poster bed with a trapeze bar on one end and a variety of springs, straps, poles, and bars. For purpose of the wedding workout, only a sampling of Pilates mat exercises are included.

A popular style of class today that you will find in many studios or fitness centers is a fusion class that blends one or more mind-body styles of training. One blend that works very well is the combination of yoga and Pilates exercises, given their shared heritage.

Yoga and Pilates both place emphasis on your "core" muscles—your abdominals, lower back, and dozens of small spinal muscles. When all of those small, internal muscles are optimally strong, they lend support, stability, and added strength to your weight training activities. Your aerobic exercises also benefit because the more you can stabilize your posture, the more you can access the strength and power in your legs and arms, due to a more efficient transfer of force through your body.

The regular practice of Pilates provides the following benefits for healthy participants:

- Improved posture
- Stronger abdominal and back muscles
- Stronger pelvic and shoulder stabilizer muscles
- Balanced muscle development
- Improved breathing
- Better coordination and balance
- Reduced likelihood of back pain or injury
- Enhanced confidence and self-esteem
- Improved mind-body connection if practiced with focused attention
- Superior athletic performance

Because of the broad spectrum of benefits that can be derived from Pilates practice, enthusiasts range from people who are recovering from musculoskeletal injuries to elite athletes.

Sample Pilates Mat Exercises

The Pilates mat exercises described below provide you with a small taste of the more than 500 possible exercises in the complete Pilates repertoire, which includes a variety of equipment training options. You can enjoy these few moves as part of your core training and postural improvement. If you want to learn more, look for a qualified instructor in your neighborhood. If you don't have time to explore further before your wedding, keep it on your list for something to check out when your life falls into a more regular routine.

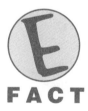

Pilates is among the fastest growing exercise programs in the fitness industry. Participation in the United States has increased more than 500 percent in the last five years. Pilates is particularly popular among models, actors, and athletes who want to focus on postural improvement.

ROLL DOWN TO PUSH UP

Figures 13-17 and 13-18
The Pilates pushup is a blended move that begins and ends in a standing position that combines stretching the entire back with strengthening the chest, back, shoulders, and arms, as well as the core muscles.

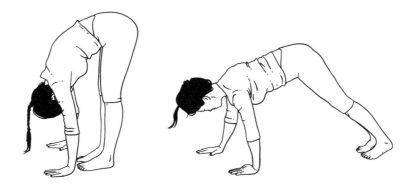

GET SET Begin in a standing position with feet hip-width apart and arms straight at your sides.

ACTION Lower your upper body head first toward the ground as you round your back until your hands reach the ground. Bend your knees, if necessary. (**SEE FIGURE 13-17**.) Walk your hands out until your hands are under your shoulders in a pushup position. (**SEE FIGURE 13-18**.) Do three to five pushups. Walk your hands back in toward your feet and round up into a standing position.

WEDDING WORKOUT POINTERS Exhale as you lower your head toward the ground. Breathe normally as you walk your hands out. Exhale as you lower into your pushups, inhale as you lift. Breathe normally as you walk your hands back in. Exhale as you round up into a standing position.

THE HUNDRED

Figures 13-19 and 13-20

The hundred strengthens and tones abdominal muscles and conditions shoulder and pelvic stabilizer and neck muscles. It is a signature Pilates mat exercise and is known for its invigorating and energizing qualities.

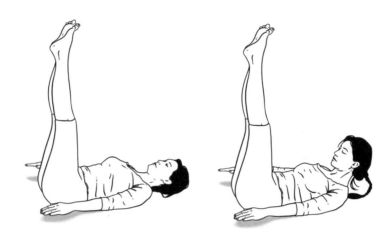

GET SET Lie on your back, with your arms straight at your sides. Bend your knees above hips, and extend one leg straight up. Lower your back into the ground for support and lift your other leg. Re-establish a level pelvic position. (**SEE FIGURE 13-19**.)

ACTION Exhale as you curl up your upper body, reaching arms forward at shoulder height, and contract your abdominals. Pump arms up and down five times as you inhale. Pump arms up and down five times as you exhale. (**SEE FIGURE 13-20**.) Repeat for ten breath cycles. The ten arm beats times ten breath cycles equals one hundred arm pumps, which is where this exercise gets its name. Avoid arching your back. Keep your abdominals tight.

WEDDING WORKOUT POINTERS If you have any neck pain or discomfort, try supporting the head with one hand, elbow pointing out with upper arm as flat as possible to keep chest open. Perform beats with other arm. Switch hands after five breath cycles.

VARIATIONS

(EASIER) Instead of keeping your legs straight, bend your knees above your hips at a 90 degree angle.

(EASIER) Keep your feet flat on the ground with your knees bent at a ninety-degree angle.

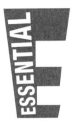

You don't have to be a serious athlete or a flexible person to excel at yoga or Pilates. If you're new, start with a beginner class. With dedicated and continued practice, it won't be long before you see results. Even if you've always thought of yourself as clumsy, you'll be amazed to see the poses and exercises you can master!

LEG PULL, FACING UP

Figures 13-21 and 13-22

The leg pull, facing up, strengthens and tones shoulders, arms, buttocks, and thighs. It conditions shoulder, spinal, and pelvic stabilizer muscles and stretches the hamstrings. It is an advanced exercise.

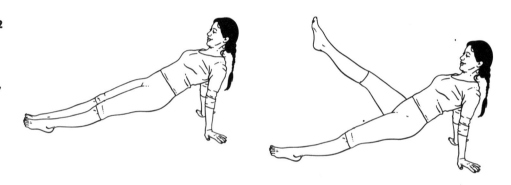

GET SET Sit with legs straight and palms down behind and outside your hips, fingers facing whichever direction is comfortable.

ACTION Push your heels into the ground as you squeeze your buttocks and lift your hips and torso upward into a reverse plank position. Stabilize your shoulders by sliding them back and down. Look ahead. (**SEE FIGURE 13-21**.) Exhale as you lift one leg as high as you can while keeping a solid plank position. (**SEE FIGURE 13-22**.) Inhale as you lower your leg. Repeat two more times. Repeat with the other leg.

WEDDING WORKOUT POINTERS Squeeze your buttocks and tighten your abdominals to prevent sagging at the hips.

VARIATIONS

Instead of doing all three lifts on one leg and then lifting the other, alternate lifting each leg for three rounds.

(EASIER) Simply hold the reverse plank position for thirty seconds without adding the leg lifts if you are unable to stabilize the plank position.

(EASIER) Keep knees bent and feet on mat and lift up into a reverse tabletop position. Hold for thirty seconds. When you get stronger, work up to the reverse plank and eventually to the leg pull, facing up.

LEG PULL, FACING DOWN

Figures 13-23 and 13-24
The leg pull, facing down strengthens, and tones shoulders, arms, buttocks, and thighs. It conditions shoulder, spinal, and pelvic stabilizer muscles. It is an advanced exercise.

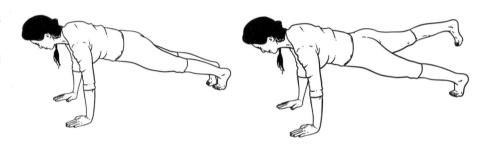

GET SET Kneel on all fours on the floor. Walk your hands forward until your hands are slightly more than shoulder-width apart and your torso resembles a slanted board. Tighten your abdominal and buttock muscles to support your lower back. Push up onto the balls of your feet into pushup position. **(SEE FIGURE 13-23.)**

ACTION Exhale as you lift one leg with your foot flexed. Keep good posture. **(SEE FIGURE 13-24.)** Inhale as you lower leg back to ground. Repeat two times.

WEDDING WORKOUT POINTERS If wrist pressure makes it uncomfortable to do this exercise, try doing this exercise with your elbows bent and forearms resting on the ground. Place your elbows directly under your shoulders.

VARIATIONS

Instead of doing all three lifts on one leg and then the other, lift alternate legs for three rounds.

Chapter 14

Starting with Basic Workouts

Now comes the nitty gritty of shaping up for your wedding. All the exercises and training principles that you need have been described. In this chapter, everything is put together into a comprehensive program to get you feeling and looking your best. You'll start building your cardio base, toning your muscles, stretching to work out kinks, and improving your posture and body awareness. Start at the beginning, build gradually, and by the time your wedding arrives, you'll be ready to dance the night away!

Walking for Weight Loss and Wellness

Let's begin by building your cardiovascular endurance or your aerobic fitness. One of the best exercises to improve your health and fitness is walking. Walking is the body's most natural form of movement. It has a low risk of injury, is easy to fit into your day, is inexpensive, and it delivers powerful results. Study after study confirms that people who walk regularly have lower risks of disease and higher levels of health. Walking is something you can enjoy all through your life. And, you can easily begin with a few minutes at a time and work up to walking a marathon if that is one of your goals.

Walking Means Fitness for Life

The most important benefits of walking are its convenience and its power to improve health and shape you up. You can walk indoors or outdoors, at any time of day, and in any type of weather. You can walk alone or use the time to catch up with friends, spend quality moments with a pet, or even to conduct business. You can use it to enhance your leisure activities like when you play golf or go hiking, or you can simply do it as a way to stay in shape and to release stress. Studies show that walking consistently helps you to:

- Maintain a healthy weight
- Increase metabolism
- Reduce stress and tension
- Improve mood and feelings of well-being
- Increase muscle mass and burn fat mass
- Strengthen the heart muscle
- Improve the functioning of your circulatory system
- Strengthen bones
- Improve joint health
- Boost energy
- Improve sleep
- Lower risks of injury

- Tone muscles for a firm and fit appearance
- Lengthen life

All you need to do is lace up your sneakers and begin.

Walking for Your Wedding Workout Program

Your wedding workout program is based on a walking program to improve your cardiovascular fitness. If you enjoy other aerobic activities such as swimming, cycling, running, or cross-country skiing, that's great. Feel free to substitute those activities for the walking programs that are described. Because walking is the easiest, most economical, and most widely accessible aerobic activity for all people, this workout is based on a walking program.

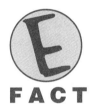

FACT

Moderate intensity walking on a daily basis is the most effective way for people to lose weight and keep it off. This is based on data from the National Weight Control Registry, which tracks people who have been able to lose at least 10 percent or more of their body weight and keep it off for more than five years.

Keep in mind that walking is not for wimps. Walking, while suitable for people who are older, is also an activity that can be tremendously challenging. Many people have lost hundreds of pounds successfully through consistent walking. If you haven't been a walking enthusiast before, give it a try. You may find that the pleasure and variety of walking daily is so great, that you'll soon be hooked as are millions of other Americans.

In fact, more than seventy million Americans walk for fitness and health. More and more parks and recreation centers are improving walking paths and accessibility to encourage more physical activity. Check your local community events to find walk-friendly paths and whether organized walks are being offered.

What to Wear

Walking is fortunately an economical activity. Your most important and significant investment is in the shoes that you wear. Take time to find a comfortable, sturdy shoe that fits the needs of your foot and provides good arch support. Shoe technology these days is quite sophisticated. Go to a reputable athletic footwear store that allows returns if the shoe is not a good fit for you. While this may cost a few more dollars initially, you will benefit from this personal attention during your first purchase. Once you know the brand and size that works for you, you can look for more economical options (such as ordering online).

If you plan to walk both at home and at the office, consider investing in two pairs of shoes. This way you can always leave a pair at work. Otherwise, you will have to carry your shoes daily. It's important to make getting active as easy as possible. Again, while this represents a bigger investment in the beginning, it will pay multiple dividends over time in your improved health and quality of life.

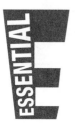

Buy shoe inserts. Today's shoes do not come with insoles that last as long as the outer parts of the shoes, but the cushioning that provides you with support is essential for comfort. When you purchase your shoes, ask the salesperson to also help you to find an appropriate insole. This will make a tremendous difference in your long-term comfort.

When purchasing walking sportswear, look for fabrics that breathe. Many modern fabrics also feature wicking qualities that actually draw your perspiration away from your skin. This can definitely enhance your walking comfort. Be sure to wear an athletic sports bra. Comfort is your primary objective. Wear bright colors to make sure that you are visible to any traffic. You can purchase reflector vests as well that improve your visibility.

Sun protection is also important. Be sure to wear sunscreen. Hats are also a good idea to protect your face. Depending on how sensitive you are to sun exposure, you may want to purchase a hat that also shields the back of your neck. Sunglasses provide coverage for your eyes. Choose a lightweight and comfortable pair. More than anything, you want your time during your walks to be as enjoyable as possible. Find accessories that work best for you. For more detailed information on clothing and accessories, review Chapter 2.

A Pedometer

While it's not necessary to purchase a pedometer, it's a great tool to measure your progress and keep you motivated. Studies show that if you take 10,000 steps on most days of the week, you'll realize many health benefits. These steps do not have to be performed at a particular intensity level or for a specific duration. What they represent is that you have maintained a level of daily activity that contributes to your health.

Wearing a pedometer motivates you because it helps you monitor exactly how much you move around during the day. If you've had a busy, active day, you can supplement that with a short walk to reach your daily goal. If your day has been fairly inactive, then you can save time for a longer walk. This can help you to become more active every day, which makes a significant difference in your overall calorie burn as well as your health and well-being. Studies show that wearing a pedometer causes people to move more and to lose weight successfully.

A Water Bottle

Staying properly hydrated is essential for good health. If you are taking short walks, it's not necessary to carry a water bottle with you. However, if you're going for walks that are longer than an hour, it's a good idea to either bring your own water or choose a route that goes by water fountains. Some companies create belt packs that serve as water bottle carriers that are handy for longer walks. Most important, remember to drink plenty of fluids before and after your walk, as well as during your walk.

Walking Warm-Up

You can walk indoors at a shopping mall or on a treadmill. You can walk outdoors through your neighborhood or at local parks or schools. Regardless of where you walk, you need to warm up your body to prepare it for getting active. When you first start out, start at a comfortable pace. Let your arms hang naturally at your sides and swing rhythmically with each step. Stand up as tall as you can and maintain good posture.

After about five minutes of walking, if you enjoy performing some stretches to make your walk more comfortable, you can. Do not hold the stretches for more than ten to twenty seconds, however, because you do not want to cool down and lose the benefits of your warm-up. After you complete your stretches, continue with your walk.

Walking Technique

Posture is the most important aspect of walking technique. Stand tall with your ears in line with your shoulders, arms at your sides, shoulders above hips, and abdominal muscles slightly pulled in to actively support your lower back. If you want to increase the intensity of your walk, bend your elbows at a ninety-degree angle, and swing your arms more vigorously. Take more steps, rather than longer strides. Hold your head upright rather than down to maintain good posture. If you need to look at the ground, lower your eyes, instead of your entire head. Strike heel first and push forward through the ball of your foot, actively using all your leg muscles. Keep your elbows in at your sides. Avoid swinging your arms across your body.

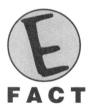

FACT

Meditation can help you keep yourself from being stressed about your wedding while you're walking. If you can't stop your constant flurry of thoughts, a little mental discipline is in order. Meditation will help you to quiet the internal chatter and get a handle on things so you can focus on your priorities and accomplish more.

Walking Cool Down

After you finish the brisk part of your walk, take time to slowly bring your body back to the way it felt when you began. Relax your breathing and calm your heart rate. You only need to spend a few minutes on your walking cool down, but be sure to take this time.

After your walk is a great time to include some final stretches. Unlike the beginning of your walk, your muscles are warm and ready to enjoy a long stretch. Breathe deeply and hold each stretch anywhere from twenty to thirty seconds. A good rule of thumb is to hold each stretch for at least three deep breath cycles. A breath cycle equals one inhalation and one exhalation. Enjoy your stretches and your feeling of accomplishment. You've just made a great positive effort to enhance your health. Enjoy the moment and feel good about yourself.

Your Walking Workouts

When you first start walking, go ahead and break up your workouts into several small workouts during the day. This helps you to increase your conditioning gradually and allows you to fit it easily into your day. If your goal is simply to improve your health, research substantiates that as little as thirty minutes a day is sufficient activity to get results. You can even split that time into three ten-minute bouts.

Building a Base

For the first two months, your goal when you start aerobic training is to build a conditioning base. The following is a progressive six-week program that gradually increases in difficulty each week. If you reach a point where you feel that it's too much, then repeat the prior week's program until you feel ready to challenge the next level of difficulty. For weeks seven and eight, simply repeat week six until you can comfortably complete the fifty-five minute to one hour walk.

Many of the walks are broken up into shorter walks throughout the day because you're likely to be so busy with all of your wedding preparations and other commitments that you'll have a hard time getting started with your exercise. The biggest reason people fail to exercise is because they believe they don't have time. You can find time for ten minutes, and even a ten-minute walk is better than no walk. Also, breaking up your walking throughout the day gives your metabolism periodic bursts for more calorie burning.

Remember that increasing your lifestyle activity as discussed in Chapter 3 is critically important—do these walks as part of your normal schedule. For example, park further away or get off the commuter train one stop earlier so that you can complete two of your twenty-minute walks when you travel to and from the office. Do extra laps around the grocery store to fit in a ten-minute walk. Be creative and add more steps at every available chance throughout the day *and* brainstorm even more ways to create additional walking opportunities.

Table 14-1

Beginning 6- to 8-Week Walking Program						
Week	**Mon**	**Tues**	**Wed**	**Thurs**	**Fri**	**Sat**	**Sun**
1	1–3 10-min walks	Rest or 10-min walk	1–3 10-min walks	Rest or 10-min walk	1–3 10-min walks	Rest or 10-min walk	1 20-min walk and 1 10-min walk
2	1 15-min walk	2 15-min walks	Rest or 1 15-min walk	2 20-min walks	1 10- to 15-min walk	1 20-min walk and 1 25-min walk	Rest
3	1 25-min walk and 1 15-min walk	1 15-min walk	2 20-min walks	1 10–15-min walk or rest	1 30-min walk	Rest	1 35-min walk
4	1 15-min walk	2 20-min walks	1 15-min walk	1 30-min walk and 1 20-min walk	Rest or 1 10–15-min walk	1 35-min walk	1 30-min walk or 2 15-min walks
5	1 25-min walk and 1 20-min walk	1 10–20-min walk	2 20-min walks	1 15–20-min walk	3 15-min walks	Rest	1 45-min walk
6	3 20-min walks	1 15–25-min walk	1 35-min walk	Rest	1 55–60-min walk	Rest or 1 15-20-min walk	1 30-min walk

Setting Your Walking Pace

When it comes to setting your walking pace, start with what you can do comfortably today and increase your ability to walk more quickly as your conditioning improves. To learn how to judge pace, time yourself as you walk around a track for four laps. This will give you your one mile per hour pace. An alternative way to measure your pace is to count how many steps that you take in one minute, and compare with the categories below. The following are four progressive pace levels:

1. **Easy Stroll:** Slower than three miles per hour, which is greater than a twenty-minute mile pace. This is fewer than 105 steps per minute.
2. **Health Walk:** At least three miles per hour, which equals a twenty-minute per mile pace. This is approximately 105 steps per minute.
3. **Fitness Walk:** At least four miles per hour, which equals a fifteen-minute per mile pace. This is approximately 140 steps per minute. You should break a light sweat.
4. **Power or Race Walk:** At least five miles per hour, which equals a twelve-minute per mile pace. This is approximately 175 steps per minute. You should be sweating.

Depending on your level of fitness, you may not be able to walk at a faster pace from the beginning of your program. Do your best and increase the briskness of your walk as your fitness improves. For every workout, start out and cool down with at least five minutes of easy strolling. If weight loss is a goal, work up to a minimum of a health walk pace for sixty minutes each day. The good news is that this can be broken up into several short walks and still achieve the same weight loss results.

Total Body Resistance Training Workouts

When you start weight training, similar to aerobic training, you want to build a conditioning base for the first two months. Always remember to warm up with at least five minutes of rhythmic activity such as walking, marching in place, jumping rope, or stationary cycling to increase your circulation, warm up your muscles, gradually elevate your heart rate, and warm up your joints. Cool down after every workout with gentle stretching or low-intensity exercises.

Deciding whether to train two or three days per week depends on how much time you have available and how quickly you want to see results. If you train three times per week, you will see a difference sooner. The following workouts give you choices between a longer workout (see Table 14-2) and a minimal workout (see Table 14-3) when you only have ten or fifteen minutes to spare. You don't want to always do quick workouts. But, when you're busy, something is always better than nothing, and consistency is critically important to achieve the best results.

A third training approach is to do two total body conditioning workouts (see Table 14-2) each week and one ab blaster workout (see Table 14-4), for a total of three training sessions. This program targets the weaker muscles of your core with a focused program on one day of the week to complement the other two total body programs. If you're interested in flattening your abdominal area and improving posture for your wedding day, this is the approach for you.

Start out with one set for each of the exercises. If you feel that you have more energy and can do more, try two sets. Work your way up to performing three sets of each exercise before you consider increasing the resistance level.

Table 14-2: 8-Week Basic Total Body Conditioning Workout	
Muscle Group	**Exercise**
Buttocks, Hips, Thighs	Squat and Lunge
Legs	Calf Raise and Toe Tap
Chest	Pushup and Incline Chest Press
Back	Lat Pull Down and Rhomboid Squeeze
Shoulders	Overhead Press, Side Raise, and Rear Shoulder Fly
Arms	Reverse Biceps Curl and Triceps Pushup
Abdominals	Crunch and Bicycle
Core	Plank, Back Extension and Side Plank

Table 14-3: Busy Day 15-Minute Total Body Quick Workout

Muscle Group	Exercise
Buttocks, Hips, Thighs	Squats
Chest	Pushup
Back	Lat Pull Down
Shoulders	Overhead Press
Abdominals and Core	Crunch and Bicycle

Table 14-4: Ab Blaster and Posture Workout

Muscle Group	Exercise
Core	Pelvic Tilt, Bridge, and Plank
Abdominals	Crunch and Bent Knee Side Crunch
Chest and Core	Pushup
Abdominals	Reverse Crunch and Oblique Crunch
Core	Back Extension and Side Plank
Buttocks, Hips, Thighs	Leg Press Bridge
Abdominals	Bicycle
Buttocks, Hips, Thighs	Bent Knee Rear Leg Lift
Core	Heel Dip and Reverse Plank

Stretching Routines

You can incorporate your stretching routines at the end of your cardio-training or resistance training workouts, or you can do it independently simply to relieve muscular tension and stress. Try to do individual stretches each hour throughout the day on a daily basis. For example, when you're sitting at your desk, take a break and do the seated chest and shoulder stretch or the seated triceps and back stretch. The more frequently you do stretches, the more limber you'll become.

The following stretch routine incorporates both stretching exercises and yoga exercises.

Table 14-5: Total Body Stretching Routine	
Muscle Group	**Exercise**
Back	Cat Stretch
Buttocks, Hips and Back	Knee Hug Stretch
Thighs and Legs	Lying Hamstring Stretch
Total Body	Lying Shoulder, Chest and Torso Twist Stretch
Thighs and Legs	Side-Lying Hip Flexors and Quadriceps Stretch
Buttocks and Back	Deep Buttocks Stretch
Total Body	Full Length Torso Crescent Stretch

Core Training with Yoga and Pilates

As a complement to conventional weight training, yoga and Pilates are excellent sources of total body conditioning. Instead of doing the ab blaster workout (see Table 14-4), you can substitute one combination yoga and Pilates routine. The wedding workout program is designed to provide you with a variety of choices so that you can do the workouts that are most comfortable and appealing to you.

Table 14-6: Combination Yoga, Pilates, and Core Routine
Exercise
Standing Posture Check
Deep Breathing
Squats
Roll Down to Pushup
Triceps Pushup
Child Posture with Extended Arms

Child Posture	
Cat Stretch	
All Fours Spinal Stabilization	
Cat Stretch	
Pelvic Tilt	
Bridging	
Knee Hug Stretch	
Plank	
The Hundred	
Full Length Torso Crescent Stretch	
Back Extension	
Cat Stretch	
Child Posture	
Rolling Back	

Pulling It Together—A Sample Week

Don't be overwhelmed by all of your exercise choices. Work at your own pace and increase your amount of exercise as you feel that you can handle it. Start with the walking workout to begin building your conditioning. Add in the resistance training either at the same time, or when you feel ready to begin muscle toning. Stick with these basic conditioning workouts for the first two to four months. When you feel ready to advance to harder levels of exercise, move on to the programs in Chapter 15.

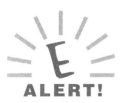

If you have any back discomfort, you want to avoid impact and avoid rapid twisting movements. Aerobic exercises to consider include walking, cycling, aqua aerobics or swimming. If you want to exercise indoors, you can try stationary cycling, treadmill walking, cross-country skiing on a Nordic track machine, or using an elliptical trainer.

To give you an idea of how all of these workouts fit together into a weekly program, Table 14-7 shows a sample schedule.

Table 14-7: Sample Basic Conditioning Weekly Schedule			
Day of Week	**Cardio-Training**	**Toning**	**Stretching**
Monday	Walk	Total body conditioning	Total body stretching
Tuesday	Walk	Rest	Individual stretches
Wednesday	Walk	Total body conditioning	Total body stretching
Thursday	Walk	Rest	Individual stretches
Friday	Walk	Ab blaster or yoga, Pilates, core routine	Total body stretching
Saturday	Rest or easy walk	Rest	Individual stretches
Sunday	Walk	Rest or individual core exercises	Individual stretches

Work at your own pace. You will benefit by adding in more core or yoga and Pilates exercises or stretching on a daily basis, but it's not essential. Listen to your body and incorporate the exercises that feel good to you into your daily schedule. You'll soon be amazed by the transformation that you begin to experience in body, mind, and spirit.

Chapter 15

Intermediate Workouts Before the Big Day

Congratulations! Now that you've built your conditioning base, you're ready to step up your program. One of the great aspects of fitness is that slow and steady training delivers results. During any individual workout, you may not feel a difference, but a few months go by and before you know it, you're feeling stronger, more energetic, toned, and your clothes are fitting differently. You're seeing results and getting hooked. Now you just have to continue on this path of healthy living.

15

Measuring Your Progress

Before you increase the level of difficulty of your program, take the time to measure your progress. Often, it's easy to forget that what you can now do easily, you weren't able to do before. Go back to Chapter 1 and repeat your assessments. This is important for two reasons: first, you can see the improvements that you have made; and second, you can confirm that you're ready to step up your training.

Staying Injury-Free

Keeping your program safe and injury-free is the top priority. You want to be able to enjoy every moment of your wedding and honeymoon. One of the most common causes of injury is doing too much exercise too soon. By repeating your assessments and confirming your progress, you're not only motivating yourself to keep going, but you're also ensuring that you're ready to work harder.

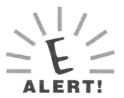

ALERT!

Before increasing your training level, it's important to have a conditioning base of at least two to six months. This ensures that your muscles and joints are conditioned and ready for higher levels of stress. Your conditioning base provides enough time for you to perfect your training skills and technique, so that as you do more difficult exercises, you remain injury free.

Checking Your Priorities

After you repeat your assessments, take a moment to consider what your leading priority or your primary training goal is before your wedding date. Your conditioning base provides overall improvement in your aerobic fitness, muscular strength and endurance, flexibility, core stability, balance, and posture. Now, you need to determine what your main objective is before your wedding date arrives.

Identifying your primary goal is important to focus your training. For example, you may be happy with the improvements that you've achieved, but want to continue to lose more body fat. Alternatively, you may want to focus on more muscular definition. Some women prefer simply to have toned muscles while others prefer to have very defined muscles. Or, depending on your condition before you started training, you may want to continue improving your posture, so that standing tall without a slouch becomes your natural stance at all times.

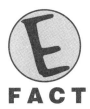

FACT

It's common for people to want to improve both muscular strength and endurance, or, in other words, to improve both muscle size and definition and tone. Most effective training, however, is the result of focusing specifically on one aspect per training quarter. This is known as periodization.

This chapter includes workouts to boost your cardio-training, raise the intensity of your muscle conditioning, further refine your postural training, and deepen your mind-body connection. Depending on what you have decided to focus upon, you may choose to emphasize one aspect of your training and continue with basic conditioning in other areas, or you can add difficulty to all aspects of your training program. It depends on what you want to achieve and how you feel. Whenever you feel that you're doing too much, simply scale back to an easier level. Learn to listen to your body and take it one day, and one workout, at a time.

Avoid all or nothing thinking. It's always better to do *something*, rather than nothing. Don't give up if you feel that some of these workouts are too difficult. Go back and continue to build your base level of conditioning. Remember that your workouts are time and space for you to take care of yourself and to burn off steam from your other pressures. Do not let your training time become a source of stress. Keep it as a source of pleasure and stress relief.

Attaining Your Goal Level of Fitness

If weight loss is your primary goal, focus on developing your cardio-fitness and increasing the amount of aerobic exercise that you do each week. If firming up your muscles and seeing more muscle tone is your main objective, focus on improving your muscular endurance. If increasing your muscle size and definition is your primary desire, then focus on upping your muscular strength. If working on posture is the ultimate area that you need to improve, focus on core training, yoga, and Pilates.

When you focus on a particular aspect of fitness, it does not mean that you discontinue training the other components. What it means is that you can increase the level of the work that you do in that one domain. Keep up your fitness gains in the other areas by sticking with the basic conditioning program. Most important, and this cannot be overemphasized, listen to your body.

Stepping Up Your Cardio with Intervals

Interval training is a great, fun, and time efficient way to increase the intensity of your walking workouts. What's great about doing intervals is that you work at a higher intensity, but only in short bursts. You don't have to be able to sustain that harder stage of work for long periods of time. This allows you to stimulate your system for better conditioning and gradually work up to more difficult levels.

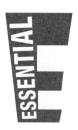

Interval training is a more advanced form of cardio-training. Start an interval training program only after you've established a solid base of aerobic fitness. For easier aerobic intervals, work at 60 to 80 percent of max heart rate. For advanced intervals, challenge your anaerobic threshold by working at 80 to 90 percent.

Interval training is fun because it offers variety to your program. Because interval training is more intense, you're not going to do it every day. Instead, you'll do it two to three times per week. With your other workouts, you will increase your time, distance, and frequency of your walking to keep pushing up the work load.

Lastly, interval training is efficient. For the same amount of time that you would take to walk at a steady pace, when you add in interval training, you use more energy or burn more calories. For the same amount of time, you're working harder. Therefore, on particularly busy days, interval training is a great way to maintain the higher state of conditioning that you've developed in the same amount of time.

Here are some sample interval training workouts:

Table 15-1: Interval Workout I–30 minutes	
Warm up for 5 minutes with an easy stroll	
Increase intensity to a health walk for 5 minutes	
Interval Intensity and Length	**Recovery**
Fitness walk for 30 seconds	Health walk for 30 seconds
Fitness walk for 45 seconds	Health walk for 45 seconds
Fitness walk for one minute	Health walk for one minute
Fitness walk for one minute	Health walk for one minute
Fitness walk for one minute	Health walk for one minute
Fitness walk for 45 seconds	Health walk for 45 seconds
Fitness walk for 30 seconds	Health walk for 30 seconds
Cool down for 5 minutes with an easy stroll	
End with standing stretches for 5 minutes	

To increase the level of difficulty of this workout, replace each health walk with a fitness walk and replace each fitness walk with a power walk. To increase the length of the workout, add more intervals.

Table 15-2: Interval Workout II—35 minutes

Warm up for 5 minutes with an easy stroll

Increase intensity to a health walk for 3 minutes

Interval Intensity and Length	Recovery
Fitness walk for 30 seconds	Health walk for 30 seconds
Fitness walk for 45 seconds	Health walk for 45 seconds
Fitness walk for one minute	Health walk for one minute
Fitness walk for 90 seconds	Health walk for one minute
Fitness walk for two minutes	Health walk for one minute
Fitness walk for 150 seconds	Health walk for one minute
Fitness walk for 150 seconds	Health walk for one minute

Cool down for 5 minutes with an easy stroll

End with standing stretches for 5 minutes

To increase the level of difficulty of this workout, replace each health walk with a fitness walk, and replace each fitness walk with a power walk. To increase the length of the workout, add in more intervals.

Increasing Endurance with Longer Workouts

Long, slow distance training is another method to increase the difficulty of your aerobic exercise and to burn more energy. If you find that you really enjoy walking, you can add variety to your routines by incorporating one long walk per week. This is also a great way to manage weight and lose excess fat. You can use this time to explore a beautiful park or area in your community. Or, if you're doing a long walk on a treadmill, this can be when you watch a favorite television program.

When you increase mileage, you need to observe the following basic guidelines to avoid injury:

- Do not increase your mileage until you have established a base of walking at least 45 consecutive minutes on most days of the week.

- Increase mileage by only 10 percent per week. For example, if you're walking 15 miles per week, increase by no more than 1.5 miles, for a total of 16.5 miles the next week.
- Rest at least one day per week.
- During a one-week training plan, include two short walks, two to three medium-length walks, and one long walk.

Table 15-3 shows a sample training program that includes interval walks and distance walking.

Table 15-3: Sample Intermediate to Advanced Cardio-Training Weekly Schedule		
Day of Week	**Type of Training**	**Duration**
Monday	Interval walk	35 minutes
Tuesday	2 short walks	15 minutes
Wednesday	Interval walk	30 minutes
Thursday	2 short walks	15–20 minutes
Friday	Medium walk	40–45 minutes
Saturday	Long, slow distance walk	60 minutes
Sunday	Rest	

Now that you understand the variables that you have to work with, you can organize your walks accordingly. If you're not in the mood for interval walks, simply enjoy walking at a steady state. If you don't have time for a longer walk, break up your walking into two to three walks per day for ten to twenty minutes at a time. If weight loss is a top goal, try to walk at least one hour per day on an accumulated basis.

Weight Training Split Routines

Wedding dresses typically reveal the neck, shoulders, and décolletage. Sometimes, dresses also highlight the back. If your dress falls into any of these categories, you may want to spend more time toning your upper body.

Once you've established a conditioning base, you can start doing more exercises without undue muscle soreness. This is the time to consider split routines that involve focusing on specific muscle groups or certain parts of the body during each workout, rather than always training the entire body.

Split routines offer several benefits:

- You can do your weight training several days a week for fewer minutes at a time, rather than skipping a day in between workouts.
- You can achieve better muscular development because you can do a wider selection of exercises for each targeted muscle group.
- You can add variety to your routines, instead of doing the same total body conditioning program, two to three days a week.

Here's a sample training schedule: on Monday, train your upper body, Tuesday your lower body, and on Wednesday, rest; on Thursday, train your upper body, Friday your lower body, and on the weekend, rest. Alternatively, you can rest every other day.

The most important rule to keep in mind when doing split routines is that you should not train the same muscle group two days in a row. The challenge to observing this rule is that many exercises use more than one muscle group. This is generally avoided if you focus on upper and lower body split routines.

Table 15-4 and Table 15-5 show sample upper and lower body split routines that you can do according to the alternating day schedules described above. You don't want to train your abdominals daily, so you can choose to train them together with either your lower or upper body. In contrast, you can do core exercises that focus on stabilization on a daily basis.

Table 15-4: Sample Upper Body Split Routine	
Muscle Group	**Exercise**
Chest	Pushup, Incline Chest Press, and Chest Fly
Back	Lat Pull Down, One Arm Row, and Rhomboid Squeeze
Shoulders	Overhead Press, Side Raise, and Rear Shoulder Fly

Arms	Biceps Curl, Triceps Pushup, Reverse Biceps Curl, and Triceps Dip
Core	Plank, Side Plank, All Fours Spinal Stabilization, and Reverse Plank

Table 15-5: Sample Lower Body Split Routine

Muscle Group	Exercise
Buttocks, Hips, Thighs	Squat, Lunge, Leg Press Bridge, and Bent Knee Rear Leg Lift
Thighs	Leg Curl, Outer Thigh Leg Lift, and Inner Thigh Leg Lift
Legs	Legs, Calf Raise, and Toe Tap
Abdominals	Crunch, Reverse Crunch, Oblique Crunch, Bicycle
Core	Plank, Heel Dip, Pelvic Tilt, Bridging, and Back Extension

If improving your muscle tone is a top priority, it's a good idea to follow a split program. At the same time, if you've already decided that you want to focus on weight loss and you're going to step up your aerobic training, it's not a good idea to do too much weight training. This is where you need to make choices based on what is your main training objective.

Refer back to the discussion in Chapter 8 on body types and identifying your training goal. If you tend to build muscle easily, you may not want or need to increase the amount of your resistance training beyond the basic conditioning program. In contrast, if you're more of an ectomorph and you have a hard time getting results from your resistance training, following a split program is ideal for you. Consider who you are, how your body responds to exercise, and what results you want to see by your wedding day.

Another reason to modify your program is to keep both your mind and your body interested. If you start feeling bored with your routine, it's time to alter exercises or style to stay actively engaged. Even switching from dumbbells to resistance bands adds elements of change. It's not only your mind that loses interest. As your muscles become conditioned, unless you stimulate them in new ways, you'll reach a plateau where you're no longer seeing improvements.

Muscle Strength Versus Muscle Endurance

Another way to add diversity to your resistance training is to focus on muscular strength, size, or endurance. As you learned in Chapter 1, muscular strength and endurance are two different qualities. After you set up your conditioning base, it's good to focus your training on a specific characteristic. If you're interested in increasing muscular size, focus on multiple sets with fewer repetitions. If you're interested in improving endurance, which results in leaner muscles, do multiple sets with multiple repetitions.

Here's how to add these protocols to your training program.

To increase muscular size:

- Do 6 to 12 repetitions to failure.
- Rest for 30 to 90 seconds between each set.
- Do 3 to 6 sets of each exercise.

To increase muscular endurance:

- Do 12 to 24 repetitions to failure.
- Rest for 30 seconds or less between each set.
- Do 2 to 3 sets of each exercise.

Use these protocols in your split routines to emphasize the results that you want to achieve. If your emphasis is to increase muscular size, depending on your age and level of conditioning, it may be too intense to do two hard workouts per body area per week. Another option is to use the split routine, but do one workout with fewer reps to failure early in the week. For the second workout, do the same routine but with higher reps to failure by using a lower resistance or lighter weight. Using the ingredients in the book, you can tailor the workouts to achieve the exact results that you desire.

Ten-Minute Daily Core Training and Stretching

All body types benefit from consistent core training. In fact, the best results from core training exercises come from doing a few minutes on a daily basis, rather than a single concentrated program only once a week. When you stimulate your core muscles to support your posture, you remember to use those postural muscles more each day. That means that even when you're not exercising, you remember to stand up straight, sit tall in your chair, and correct your posture every time that you slouch.

Now that you've established your conditioning base, you can add daily core training to your routine. Table 15-6 provides a sample ten-minute core routine that you can choose to do either in the morning or in the evening. This workout combines stretching, core, yoga, and Pilates exercises for total well-being.

Table 15-6: Ten-Minute Yoga, Pilates, and Core Routine
Exercise
Pelvic Tilt
Bridging
Knee Hug Stretch
Plank
Child Posture
Crunch
Oblique Crunch
Full Length Torso Crescent Stretch
Knee Hug Stretch
All Fours Spinal Stabilization
Cat Stretch

Back Extension
Child Posture
Bicycle
Lying Shoulder, Chest, and Torso Twist Stretch

If you're too busy to do your resistance training workout, you can still find time to fit in a core workout. Combine this with your regular walking program and you will continue to experience improvements in posture and fitness. This is also a great back health program. Keep it up and find yourself healthy and pain free for a joyous wedding, reception, and honeymoon.

If you've started taking yoga or Pilates class, that's great. Go ahead and enjoy it one or two days a week. On those days, you don't need to do a resistance training program or incorporate additional stretching. Yoga and Pilates both provide muscle conditioning and stretching benefits, so there's no need to overdo it.

Continue with your daily individual stretches to reduce tension, help you to relax, and to create long, lean muscles. Either follow the routine in Chapter 14 or find creative ways to slip in stretches during your day.

Sample Weekly Schedule

The wedding workout is designed with customization in mind. These options help you to get the results that you want. You're not meant to do all the exercises described above. You're meant to pick and choose and design the workout program that focuses on the targeted areas that you want to improve. You can always fall back on the basic conditioning program if you feel that you're not ready to do more work, or you simply don't have time to step up your program.

To give you an idea of how these intermediate workouts fit together into a weekly program, Table 15-7 shows a sample schedule.

Table 15-7: Sample Intermediate Workout Weekly Schedule

Day of Week	Cardio-Training	Muscle Conditioning	Core Training	Stretching
Monday	Walk	Upper Body Split	10-minute Core	Total Body Stretching
Tuesday	Walk	Lower Body Split	10-minute Core	Individual Stretches
Wednesday	Walk	Rest	Rest	Total Body Stretching
Thursday	Walk	Upper Body Split	10-minute Core	Individual Stretches
Friday	Walk	Lower Body Split	10-minute Core	Total Body Stretching
Saturday	Rest or Easy Walk	Rest	Rest	Individual Stretches
Sunday	Walk	Rest	Rest	Individual Stretches

This sample weekly schedule is based on the assumption that you want to increase your muscular training. If your focus is on aerobic training, follow the sample walking program (see Table 15-3) and add in total body conditioning on two or three days a week. Stick with whatever emphasis you choose for at least six to eight weeks to get results from that stage of your program. After two months, either change your emphasis, or for additional variety and fine tuning, see Chapter 16.

Chapter 16

Six-Week Countdown for a Busy Bride

Well done! By now, you've been doing your best to follow an integrated wellness program of good nutrition, consistent exercise, stress management, and healthy sleep for several months. You should be feeling and looking great, with more energy and resilience to prepare for the final, exciting events to come. Your countdown program is all about self-care. You want to keep all your hard earned fitness gains and focus on feeling and looking your best for the big day.

Final Assessment for Countdown Training

It's time for your last round of evaluations before your wedding. Once again, return to Chapter 1 and revisit the assessments. Compare the difference between today and your first day of the program. Give yourself a big pat on the back for all your hard work. Wellness doesn't simply happen to people. You develop it every day by choosing health at every opportunity. Your progress is the direct result of your commitment. Savor this moment and plan a special reward for yourself—a pampering massage, spa day, or whatever encourages you to relax and feel good. You deserve it!

As you look at your assessment results, consider what you want to achieve in these last few weeks. It's likely that your schedule is going to become tighter and tighter, particularly as all the social events—luncheons, parties, receptions—start kicking into gear. Your workout time is a special luxury that you need to protect for yourself as much as possible. At the same time, you need to be realistic.

Your life is not going to be routine during this final countdown. Given the upcoming demands on your time, take a moment to brainstorm what's going to be possible for you in terms of training. Can you keep up with at least a daily walk? Can you continue to squeeze in daily stretching and toning? Can you fit in a structured workout at least two to three days a week? Now, you need to be ultraefficient with your training.

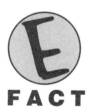

FACT

Studies show that minimal amounts of equally intense training can deter the loss of endurance and strength when insufficient time is available for longer workouts for up to four months. A minimum of two muscle conditioning sessions per week is enough to keep your toning gains.

To give you the greatest boost for your investment, the workouts in this last section focus on delivering the most results in the least amount of time. This program works because you're building on the foundation that you've already established and targeting your shape-up goals. Customize how you put together the programs set forth below depending on whether you want to focus on losing more weight or on creating more muscle tone or definition. If you've achieved the shape that you want, emphasize pure maintenance.

Pedometer Walking to Manage Weight

You have successfully incorporated aerobic exercise into your daily activities. To help you continue to manage your weight, reduce stress, and feel great, use your pedometer during this last six to eight weeks before the wedding. Wearing your pedometer helps you stay on track with a minimal amount of effort because it serves as a constant reminder of whether you've reached your daily goal. Depending on what your monitor tells you mid-day, you can adjust your schedule to include a longer walk or squeeze in a few more short walks before the end of the day.

Benefits of using a pedometer include the following:

- Convenient and easy to use
- Inexpensive
- Constant reminder of your exercise goals
- Immediate feedback on your daily activity level
- Motivating you to meet your targeted steps

The targeted daily number of steps that you want to achieve depends on what your goal is for this last training period before your wedding. If your goal is to maintain the level of fitness that you've already achieved, you need to take a minimum of 10,000 steps per day, or an average of 10,000 steps per day over a one-week period. The typical person takes approximately 2,000 steps per mile. Therefore, this means that you're going to walk approximately five miles per day.

If your goal is to continue to lose weight, then you'll need to walk more steps each day. Studies show that taking approximately 15,000 steps per day helps people to achieve weight loss and meet their healthy weight goals. To reach the 15,000 step level, you need to commit to taking a walk each day in addition to incorporating more walking during your typical activities. This may not be realistic with your current schedule, though.

Avoid putting any undue pressure on yourself during this already busy time. Keep your walking fun and enjoyable as stress relief for yourself—not another source of pressure. Use the walking programs from either Chapter 14 or 15 if you have time for structured walking workouts. If you find that your schedule is simply too demanding right now, slip in as much lifestyle activity as you can and just aim for 10,000 steps per day.

Cardio-Resistance Circuit Training

Circuit training is another way to maximize your results when you're working on maintenance and you're too busy to dedicate time to both a detailed aerobic program and a detailed weight training program. Different styles of circuit training exist. One method is to move quickly from one resistance exercise directly to another without any break other than the transition time. This increases endurance and keeps the heart rate elevated in the lower end of the aerobic training zone. With cardio-resistance circuit training, you alternate aerobic intervals between resistance training sets.

Circuit training is not the best method to maximize your strength or your aerobic fitness. However, it's a great way to target both goals in one workout. If you've already established a good aerobic base of conditioning, you can maintain your base with circuit training. If you've already built up a foundation of muscle conditioning, you can maintain your muscle tone and fitness. For this busy time in your life, circuit training may be just the solution to keep you in top shape in the minimal amount of time.

Try to fit your circuit training workout in at least two days a week. On your third muscle conditioning day, fit in an ab blaster (see Table 14-4) or core training routine. Here are sample resistance circuit and cardio-resistance circuit workouts. Do one set of ten to fifteen reps each for the upper body exercises and one set of fifteen to twenty-four reps each for the lower body and abdominal exercises. Follow the exercise order because it is designed to allow one part of the body to rest while another part of the body works.

Table 16-1: Sample Resistance Circuit Workout

Muscle Group	Exercise
Buttocks, Hips	Squat
Chest	Pushup
Back	One Arm Row
Buttocks, Hips	Leg Press Bridge
Shoulders	Overhead Press
Back	Lat Pull Down
Buttocks, Hips	Lunge
Thighs	Leg Curl
Arms	Triceps Pushup
Arms	Reverse Biceps Curl
Abdominals	Crunch and Bicycle

Depending on how much time you have, you can do this circuit two to four times.

In Table 16-2, during the cardio-intervals, march, jog, jump rope, or do knee lifts and leg curls, or jumping jacks for up to one-minute of hard work, with thirty seconds to one minute of stepping side to side of recovery, for a total of five-minutes of an aerobic interval.

Table 16-2: Sample Cardio-Resistance Circuit Workout (40 to 45 Minutes)

Muscle Group	Exercise
Aerobic interval	
Buttocks, Hips	Squat and Lunge
Back	Rhomboid Squeeze
Chest	Incline Press
Back	Lat Pull Down
Aerobic interval	

Shoulders	Overhead Press, Side Raise, and Rear Shoulder Fly
Back	One Arm Row
Aerobic interval	
Arms	Triceps Dip
Arms	Reverse Biceps Curl
Arms	Triceps Pushup
Aerobic interval	
Legs	Toe Tap
Chest, Core	Roll Down to Push Up
Abdominals	Crunch and Reverse Crunch
Core	Back Extension and Cat Stretch
Abdominals	Oblique Crunch and Bicycle
Stretches	Knee Hug Stretch, Lying Hamstring Stretch, Lying Shoulder, Chest, and Torso Twist Stretch, Side-Lying Hip Flexors and Quad Stretch, Deep Buttocks Stretch, and Full Length Torso Crescent Stretch

If you don't have enough time to do the complete workout in Table 16-2, cut out the arm exercises because you're getting arm toning benefits with your chest and back training. In addition, eliminate one aerobic interval. The total workout time is then reduced to twenty-five to thirty minutes depending on how many reps of each exercise you decide to do.

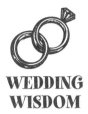

Running on a short fuse because you're overwhelmed and stretched too thin? We're often impatient and snappish at others when we don't take a break and de-stress. You might think you don't have time for relaxation, but think again. Find ways to decompress, and you'll be less likely to overreact. Then you'll have fewer arguments with your fiancé, family, and friends!

Core Training and Stretching for Posture Perfection

Keep up your ten-minute core training routine (see Table 15-6) at least three days a week and more if possible. This will continue to stimulate your postural muscles and remind you to walk tall and sit with good posture every day. You'll also want to keep up with your stretching to relieve tension and stress. Carve out time in the evening to wind down, breathe deeply, and restore your sense of inner balance.

Table 16-3 provides an evening wind down stretch routine that may come in handy during this home stretch.

Table 16-3: Evening Relaxation Stretch Routine	
Muscle Group	**Exercise**
Back, Neck, Shoulders	Cat Stretch
Back, Buttocks, Hips	Child Posture
Core	Pelvic Tilt
Core	Bridging
Back, Buttocks, Hips	Knee Hug Stretch
Total Body	Lying Shoulder, Chest, and Torso Twist Stretch

Thighs and Legs	Side-Lying Hip Flexors and Quadriceps Stretch
Buttocks and Back	Deep Buttocks Stretch
Total Body	Full Length Torso Crescent Stretch

Stretching is a feel-good exercise. Plus, stretching regularly helps to create long, lean muscles. Make time to stretch for your well-being.

Sample Weekly Schedule

During the countdown phase of your training, focus on maintenance and avoid any undue pressure on yourself. If you've done the work in prior months, now you can keep up the good work with a minimal amount of working out. It's not necessary to overdo it.

To give you an idea of how these busy bride workouts fit together into a weekly program, Table 16-4 shows a sample schedule.

Table 16-4: Sample Countdown Workout Weekly Schedule				
Day of Week	**Cardio-Training**	**Muscle Conditioning**	**Core Training**	**Stretching**
Monday	10,000 steps	Cardio-resistance circuit	Rest	P.M. stretch
Tuesday	10,000 steps	Rest	10-minute core	Individual stretches
Wednesday	10,000 steps	Cardio-resistance circuit	Rest	P.M. stretch
Thursday	10,000 steps	Rest	10-minute core	Individual stretches
Friday	10,000 steps	Rest	10-minute core	P.M. stretch
Saturday	10,000 steps	Rest	Rest	Individual stretches

| Sunday | 10,000 steps | Rest | Rest | Individual stretches |

This sample weekly schedule is based on the assumption that you're busy with pre-wedding events and planning and your workouts need to fit in as easily and smoothly as possible. If you decide that you want to do more, refer to the targeted workouts in Chapter 15. Use the elements of the wedding workout program to design your ideal training routine.

Your Bridal Portrait and Wedding Day Workout

Celebrities have long known the secret of pumping up before hitting the red carpet to give definition to muscles. When you train your muscles, you boost circulation to the targeted body part. This circulatory increase temporarily enlarges the muscle to make it more visible. If you want to enhance the definition of your cleavage, shoulders, and arms for your upcoming photo opportunities, you too can use this strategy. For tips on how to memorialize your image with "celebrity" arms, read on.

Table 16-5 is your targeted pre-bridal portrait and pre-wedding day photos workout. It's quick. It's targeted. It's for one purpose only—to help you look your best in the photos that you'll be looking at for a very long time.

Table 16-5: Pre-Wedding Photo Routine	
Muscle Group	**Exercise**
Chest	Pushup
Back	Rhomboid Squeeze
Chest	Chest Fly
Back	One Arm Row
Chest	Incline Chest Press
Back	Lat Pull Down
Chest and Back	Dumbbell Pullover

Shoulders	Overhead Press, Side Raise, and Rear Shoulder Fly
Arms	Biceps Curl, Triceps Dip, Reverse Biceps Curl, Triceps Pushup
Upper Body	Seated Triceps and Back Stretch
Upper Body	Seated Chest and Shoulder Stretch

After you do this workout, try a few deep breathing exercises. The only remaining ingredients for your photographs are your dress and your big, beautiful smile. You will treasure these memories for a lifetime.

A Toast to Your Healthy Married Life

You've done a great job in making an important commitment to your health and well-being. These habits will continue to serve you well over the course of your lifetime and enhance your married life. If you're planning to have children, being fit and strong helps you to have an easier delivery and recovery after childbirth. Living well provides you with multiple dividends and contributes to the success of your married life with your spouse.

Make an effort to continue this good work that you've accomplished as you embrace your life with your partner. You've so much to gain and absolutely nothing to lose. Living well offers you many rewards. Enjoy your life, continue to breathe deeply, and embrace health and wellness every step of the way. Congratulations!

Physical Activity Readiness Questionnaire

Physical Activity Readiness Questionnaire

Regular physical activity is fun and healthy, and increasingly more people are starting to become more active every day. Being more active is very safe for most people. However, some people should check with their doctor before they start becoming much more physically active.

The following questionnaire for people aged fifteen to sixty-nine, known as the PAR-Q or Physical Activity Readiness Questionnaire helps you determine whether you need medical supervision in your exercise program.

If you are planning to become much more physically active than you are now, start by answering the six questions. If you are over 69 years of age, and you are not used to being very active, check with your doctor regardless of your answers.

Common sense is your best guide when you answer these questions. Please read the questions carefully and answer each one honestly. Write down a *yes* or *no* response to each question.

1. Do you have a heart condition?
2. Do you feel pain in your chest when you do physical activity?
3. In the past month, have you had chest pain when you were not doing physical activity?
4. Do you have a bone or joint problem (for example, back, knee or hip) that could be made worse by a change in your physical activity?

5. Is your doctor currently prescribing drugs (for example, water pills) for your blood pressure or heart condition?
6. Do you know of any other reason why you should not do physical activity?

If you answered *yes* to one or more questions, talk with your doctor by phone or in person before you start becoming much more physically active or before you have a fitness appraisal. Tell your doctor about the PAR-Q and which questions you answered yes to.

You may be able to do any activity you want—as long as you start slowly and build up gradually. Or, you may need to restrict your activities to those that are safe for you. Talk with your doctor about the kinds of activities you wish to participate in and follow his/her advice.

If you answered *no* to all PAR-Q questions, you can be reasonably sure that you can:

- Start becoming much more physically active—begin slowly and build up gradually. This is the safest and easiest way to go.
- Take part in a fitness appraisal—this is an excellent way to determine your basic fitness so that you can plan the best way for you to live actively.

Delay becoming much more active if:

- You are not feeling well due to a temporary illness such as a cold or a fever—wait until you feel better.
- You are or may be pregnant—talk to your doctor before you start becoming more active.

If your health changes so that you then answer *yes* to any of the above questions, tell your fitness or health professional. Ask whether you should change your physical activity plan.

Chart Your Progress

Tracking Your Cardiovascular Fitness

Photocopy the log below or copy it into a training journal or your daily diary. It will help you track your progress as you count down the days to your wedding. Studies show that recording your activities helps you to meet your goals.

Walking Aerobic Fitness Test

Week 1	Date:
Location	....
Distance in number of laps	....
Time to walk 4 laps in minutes and seconds	....
Number of steps	....
Optional: Heart rate at end of test	....

Goals

Met physical activity goal of 30 minutes most days of the week ☐ YES ☐ NO

If not, what improvements to make

....

....

Notes

....

....

Week 13 Date   Date:

Location

Distance in number of laps

Time to walk 4 laps in minutes and seconds

Number of steps

Optional: Heart rate at end of test

Goals

Met physical activity goal of 30 minutes most days of the week   ❏ YES   ❏ NO

If not, what improvements to make

Notes

Week 26   Date:

Location

Distance in number of laps

Time to walk 4 laps in minutes and seconds

Number of steps

Optional: Heart rate at end of test

Goals

Met physical activity goal of 30 minutes most days of the week   ❏ YES   ❏ NO

If not, what improvements to make

Notes

Week 39	**Date:**

Location

Distance in number of laps ....

Time to walk 4 laps in minutes and seconds ....

Number of steps ....

Optional: Heart rate at end of test ....

Goals

Met physical activity goal of 30 minutes most days of the week ☐ YES ☐ NO

If not, what improvements to make

....

....

Notes

....

....

Week 52	**Date:**

Location

Distance in number of laps ....

Time to walk 4 laps in minutes and seconds ....

Number of steps ....

Optional: Heart rate at end of test ....

Goals

Met physical activity goal of 30 minutes most days of the week ☐ YES ☐ NO

If not, what improvements to make

....

....

Notes

....

....

Track Your Upper Body Strength

Photocopy the log below or copy it into a training journal or your daily diary.

Upper Body Strength Pushup Test

Week 1	Date:

Pushup variation

Number of pushups

Goals

Met strength training goal of training 2–3 days of the week   ❏ YES   ❏ NO

If not, what improvements to make

....

....

Notes

....

....

....

Week 13	Date

Pushup variation

Number of pushups

Goals

Met strength training goal of training 2–3 days of the week   ❏ YES   ❏ NO

If not, what improvements to make

....

....

Notes

....

....

....

Week 26		**Date:**	

Pushup variation ....

Number of pushups ....

Goals

Met strength training goal of training 2–3 days of the week   ❏   ❏

                                                            YES   NO

If not, what improvements to make

....

....

Notes

....

....

....

Week 39 Date		

Pushup variation ....

Number of pushups ....

Goals

Met strength training goal of training 2–3 days of the week   ❏   ❏

                                                            YES   NO

If not, what improvements to make

....

....

Notes

....

....

....

Week 52	Date:

Pushup variation ....

Number of pushups ....

Goals

Met flexibility goal of stretching 4 or more days of the week ☐ ☐
                                                YES NO

If not, what improvements to make

....

....

Notes

....

....

....

Track Your Core Fitness

Photocopy the log below or copy it into a training journal or your daily diary.

Abdominal and Core Fitness Test

Week 1	Date:

Number of situps in one minute ....

Goals

Met flexibility goal of stretching 4 or more days of the week ☐ ☐
                                                YES NO

If not, what improvements to make

....

....

Notes

....

....

....

Week 13   **Date:**

Number of sit ups in one minute ....

Goals

Met core goal of training 4 or more days of the week   ❏   ❏
                                                          YES   NO
If not, what improvements to make

....

....

Notes

....

....

....

Week 26   **Date:**

Number of sit ups in one minute ....

Goals

Met core goal of training 4 or more days of the week   ❏

If not, what improvements to make

....

....

Notes

....

....

....

Week 39   Date:

Number of sit ups in one minute

....

Goals

Met core goal of training 4 or more days of the week   ☐   ☐

                                                             YES   NO

If not, what improvements to make

....

....

Notes

....

....

....

Week 52   Date:

Number of sit ups in one minute

....

Goals

Met core goal of training 4 or more days of the week   ☐   ☐

                                                             YES   NO

If not, what improvements to make

....

....

Notes

....

....

....

Track Your Flexibility

Photocopy the log below or copy it into a training journal or your daily diary.

Week 1	Date:

Best of three attempts ....

Goals

Met flexibility goal of stretching 4 or more days of the week ❑ YES ❑ NO

If not, what improvements to make

....

....

Notes

....

....

....

Week 13	Date:

Best of three attempts ....

Goals

Met flexibility goal of stretching 4 or more days of the week ❑ YES ❑ NO

If not, what improvements to make

....

....

Notes

....

....

....

Week 26   **Date:**

Best of three attempts

....

Goals

Met flexibility goal of stretching 4 or more days of the week   ❏   ❏

If not, what improvements to make   YES   NO

....

....

Notes

....

....

....

Week 39 Date

Best of three attempts

....

Goals

Met flexibility goal of stretching 4 or more days of the week   ❏   ❏

If not, what improvements to make   YES   NO

....

....

Notes

....

....

....

Week 52 Date

Best of three attempts

....

Goals

Met flexibility goal of stretching 4 or more days of the week

       ☐   ☐

      YES   NO

If not, what improvements to make

....

....

Notes

....

....

Calculating Your Body Mass Index

The body mass index (BMI) is a measure that reduces the relationship between weight and height to one number. When you compare your BMI value to charted ranges, you get an approximation of body fatness, rather than a precise measure. The figure is not equal to a measurement of body fat percentage. The value of knowing your BMI is that it provides a rough estimate of whether your body size indicates a need to manage your weight more effectively.

To find your BMI, use the formula below, or check the Body Mass Index Chart for an approximate value. To understand what your BMI means, check the BMI categories for men and women. Overweight is defined as a BMI of 25 to 29.9; obesity is defined as a BMI equal to or more than 30.

Calculate Your BMI

To calculate your BMI, you must know your weight in pounds (measured with underwear but no shoes) and your height in inches. Follow this simple three-step method:

1. Multiply your weight by 703.
2. Divide the result by your height in inches.
3. Divide the result again by your height to get your BMI.

For example: If you are five-foot-seven (or 67 inches tall) and weigh 170 pounds, you would do the following:

1. Multiply 170×703 to get 119,510
2. Divide 119,510 by 67 to get 1,784
3. Divide 1,784 by 67 to get 26.6

In this example, the BMI is 26.6. This BMI falls in the overweight category.

Body Mass Index Chart

For a less precise answer without the math, here is a chart for men and women that gives the body mass index (BMI) for various heights (in inches) and weights (in pounds, with underwear but no shoes).

The Body Mass Index Chart										
Height					**Weight**					
4'10"	100	105	110	115	119	124	129	134	138	143	148
5'0"	107	112	118	123	128	133	138	143	148	153	158
5'1"	111	116	122	127	132	137	143	148	153	158	164
5'3"	118	124	130	135	141	146	152	158	163	169	175
5'5"	126	132	138	144	150	156	162	168	174	180	186
5'7"	134	140	146	153	159	166	172	178	185	191	198
5'9"	142	149	155	162	169	176	182	189	196	203	209
6'0"	150	157	165	172	179	186	193	200	208	215	222
6'1"	159	166	174	182	189	197	204	212	219	227	235
6'3"	168	176	184	192	200	208	216	224	232	240	248
BMI Score	**21**	**22**	**23**	**24**	**25**	**26**	**27**	**28**	**29**	**30**	**31**

The Meaning of Your BMI

BMI Scores		
18.5 to 24.9	Normal weight	Good for you! Try not to gain weight.
25 to 29.9	Overweight	Try not to gain weight, especially if your waist measurement is high. You need to manage your weight if you have two or more risk factors for heart disease.
30+	Obese	You need to manage your weight. Lose weight slowly—about half a pound to two pounds a week. See your doctor or a registered dietitian if you need help.

Resources

Health Resources

American Heart Association

National Center
7272 Greenville Avenue
Dallas, TX 75231
(800) 242-8721
www.americanheart.org

Centers for Disease Control and Prevention (CDC)

1600 Clifton Road.
Atlanta, GA 30333
Public Inquiries
(404) 639-3534 or (800) 311-3435
www.cdc.gov

The Center for Mind-Body Medicine

5225 Connecticut Avenue. N.W., Suite 414
Washington, D.C. 20015
(202) 966-7338
www.cmbm.org

National Institutes of Health
9000 Rockville Pike
Bethesda, MD 20892
(301) 496-4000
✍ *www.nih.gov*

Stanford Prevention Resource Center
Hoover Pavilion, Mail Code 5705
211 Quarry Road, Room N229
Stanford, CA 94305-5705
(650) 723-6254
✍ *http://prevention.stanford.edu*

Food and Nutrition Resources

American Dietetic Association (ADA)
120 S. Riverside Plaza, Suite 2000
Chicago, IL 60606-6995
(800) 877-1600
✍ *www.eatright.org*

Consumer Nutrition Information Line of the American Dietetic Association
To find a registered dietitian, contact the association by phone or e-mail:
(800) 366-1655
E-mail: hotline@eatright.org

Center for Science in the Public Interest
Publishes the *Nutrition Action Newsletter*
1875 Connecticut Avenue., NW, Suite 300
Washington, D.C. 20009
(202) 332-9110
E-mail: cspi@cspinet.org
✍ *www.cspinet.org*

Earthbound Farm

1721 San Juan Highway

San Juan Bautista, CA 95045

(800) 690-3200

✑ *www.ebfarm.com*

The United States Department of Agriculture

Food and Nutrition Information Center

10301 Baltimore Avenue, Room 105

Beltsville, MD 20705

(301) 504-5714

✑ *www.nal.usda.gov/fnic/*

Horizon Organic (organic dairy)

P.O. Box 17577

Boulder, CO 80308-7577

(888) 494-3020

✑ *www.horizonorganic.com*

The National Directory of Farmers Markets

Online Market Locator

✑ *www.ams.usda.gov*

The Organic Trade Association

P.O. Box 547

Greenfield, MA 01302

(413) 774-7511

E-mail: info@ota.com

✑ *www.ota.com*

Prather Ranch (organic beef)

Macdoel, CA

(877) 570-2333

E-mail: sales@PratherRanch.com

✑ *www.pratherranch.com*

Revival Doctor-Formulated Soy
1031 E. Mountain Street, Building 302
Kernersville, NC 27284
(800) 738-4825
E-mail: customercare@revivalsoy.com
www.revivalsoy.com

Trader Joe's
www.traderjoes.com

U.S. Department of Agriculture (USDA)
1400 Independence Avenue, S.W.
Washington, D.C. 20250
(202) 720-2791
Fax: (202) 720-2166
www.usda.gov

U.S. Department of Health and Human Services (HHS)
200 Independence Avenue, S.W.
Washington, D.C. 20201
(877) 696-6775
www.dhhs.gov

U.S. Food and Drug Administration (FDA)
5600 Fishers Lane
Rockville, MD 20857-0001
(888) 463-6332
www.fda.gov

Weight-Control Information Network
One Win Way
Bethesda, MD 20892-3665
(877) 946-4627
www.niddk.nih.gov

Whole Foods Market, Inc.
Research and Support Team
700 Lavaca Street, Suite 500
Austin, TX 78701
Corporate office: (512) 477-4455
⋻ *www.wholefoods.com*

Exercise Resources

American College of Sports Medicine (ACSM)
P.O. Box 1440
Indianapolis, IN 46206-1440
(317) 637-9200
⋻ *www.acsm.org*

American Council on Exercise (ACE)
4851 Paramount Drive
San Diego, CA 92123
(858) 279-8227
⋻ *www.acefitness.org*

Aquatic Exercise Association (AEA)
3439 Technology Drive, Unit 6
Nokomis, FL 34275
(888) AEA-WAVE
⋻ *www.aeawave.com*

The Cooper Institute
12330 Preston Road
Dallas, TX 75230
(972) 341-3200
⋻ *www.cooperinst.org*

IDEA Health & Fitness Association
10455 Pacific Center Court
San Diego, CA 92121-4339
(800) 999-4332, Ext. 7
✎ *www.ideafit.com*

International Health, Racquet & Sportsclub Association (IHRSA)
263 Summer Street
Boston, MA 02210
(800) 228-4772
E-mail: info@ihrsa.org
✎ *http://cms.ihrsa.org*

National Strength and Conditioning Association (NSCA)
1885 Bob Johnson Drive
Colorado Springs, CO 80906
(800) 815-6826
✎ *http://nsca-lift.org*

Department of Health and Human Services
President's Council on Physical Fitness and Sports (PCPFS)
200 Independence Avenue, S.W., Room 738-H
Washington, D.C. 20201-0004
(202) 690-9000
✎ *www.fitness.gov*

YMCA of the USA
101 N. Wacker Drive
Chicago, IL 60606
(888) 333-9622 or (800) 872-9622
Fax: (312) 977-0031
✎ *www.ymca.net*

Disabled Sports Organizations

**The National Center on Physical Activity
and Disability**
Department of Disability and Human Development
University of Illinois at Chicago
1640 W. Roosevelt Road
Chicago, IL 60608-6904
(800) 900-8086
E-mail: ncpad@uic.edu
✍ *www.ncpad.org*

Disabled Sports, USA (DSUSA)
451 Hungerford Drive, #100
Rockville, MD 20850
(301) 217-0960
✍ *www.dsusa.org*

Rehabilitation Institute of Chicago
Helen M. Galvin Center for Health
and Fitness
710 N. Lake Shore Drive, 3rd Floor
Chicago, IL 60611
(312) 238-5001
✍ *www.rehabchicago.org*

Dog Walking Resources

The Humane Society of the United States
2100 L Street, N.W.
Washington, D.C. 20037
(202) 452-1100
✍ *www.hsus.org*

The American Society for the Prevention of Cruelty to Animals
Find a shelter in your area.
✑ *www.aspca.org*

PAWS: The Progressive Animal Welfare Society
Volunteer Dog Walker
✑ *www.paws.org/help/vol/*

Pets911
7301 E. Helm Drive, Building D
Scottsdale, AZ 85260-3139
(480) 889-2640
✑ *www.pets911.com*

Pilates and Yoga Resources

Balanced Body Pilates
8220 Ferguson Avenue
Sacramento, CA 95828
(800) 745-2837
✑ *www.pilates.com*

Pilates PhysicalMind Institute
84 Wooster Street, Suite 502
New York, NY 10012
(800) 505-1990
E-mail: info@themethodpilates.com
✑ *www.themethodpilates.com*

The Pilates Method Alliance (PMA)
P.O. Box 370906
Miami, FL 33137-0906
(886) 573-4946
E-mail: info@pilatesmethodalliance.org
✑ *www.pilatesmethodalliance.org*

Stott Pilates Merrithew Corporation
2200 Yonge Street, Suite 500
Toronto, ONT M4S 2C6
Canada
(800) 910-0001
E-mail: info@stottpilates.com
✍ *www.stottpilates.com*

Sivananda Yoga Vedanta Centres
1200 Arguello Boulevard
San Francisco, CA 94122
(415) 681-2731
Fax: (415) 681-5162
✍ *www.sivananda.org*

Yoga Alliance (YA)
7801 Old Branch Avenue, Suite 400
Clinton, MD 20735
(877) (964-2255)
E-mail: info@yogaalliance.org
✍ *www.yogaalliance.org*

YogaFit Training Systems Worldwide
811 North Catalina Avenue, Suite 1102
Redondo Beach, CA 90277
(888) 786-3111
E-mail: info@yogafit.com
✍ *www.yogafit.com*

Product Resources for Exercise

ACCUSPLIT, Stopwatch Company of the World
2290A Ringwood Avenue
San Jose, CA 95131
(800) 935-1996
E-mail: sales@ACCUSPLIT.com
www.accusplit.com

Fitness Wholesale
Fitness equipment and accessories
895-A Hampshire Road
Stow, OH 44224
(800) 537-5512
E-mail: fw@fwonline.com
www.fwonline.com

Junonia Roaman's
Fitness apparel for plus-sized women
P.O. Box 4408
Taunton, MA 02780-0433
Tel: (800) 677-0229
www.roamans.com

Marirose Charbonneau
Fitness apparel for women
(877) 866-7673 or (760) 734-4090
E-mail: marirosecharbonneau@mac.com

Polar Electro Inc.
1111 Marcus Avenue, Suite M15
Lake Success, NY 11042-1034
(800) 227-1314
E-mail: customer.service.usa@polar.fi
www.polarusa.com

Power Music

435 W. 400 South, Second Floor

Salt Lake City, UT 84101

(800) 777-2328

🖱 *www.powermusic.com*

Soundings of the Planet

P.O. Box 4472

Bellingham, WA 98227

(800) 937-3223

E-mail: peace@soundings.com

🖱 *www.soundings.com*

Index

THE EVERYTHING SERIES!

BUSINESS & PERSONAL FINANCE

Everything® **Accounting Book**
Everything® Budgeting Book
Everything® Business Planning Book
Everything® Coaching and Mentoring Book
Everything® Fundraising Book
Everything® Get Out of Debt Book
Everything® Grant Writing Book
Everything® Home-Based Business Book, 2nd Ed.
Everything® Homebuying Book, 2nd Ed.
Everything® Homeselling Book, 2nd Ed.
Everything® Investing Book, 2nd Ed.
Everything® Landlording Book
Everything® Leadership Book
Everything® **Managing People Book, 2nd Ed.**
Everything® Negotiating Book
Everything® Online Auctions Book
Everything® Online Business Book
Everything® Personal Finance Book
Everything® Personal Finance in Your 20s and 30s Book
Everything® Project Management Book
Everything® Real Estate Investing Book
Everything® Robert's Rules Book, $7.95
Everything® Selling Book
Everything® **Start Your Own Business Book, 2nd Ed.**
Everything® Wills & Estate Planning Book

COOKING

Everything® Barbecue Cookbook
Everything® Bartender's Book, $9.95
Everything® Chinese Cookbook
Everything® **Classic Recipes Book**
Everything® Cocktail Parties and Drinks Book
Everything® College Cookbook
Everything® **Cooking for Baby and Toddler Book**
Everything® Cooking for Two Cookbook
Everything® Diabetes Cookbook
Everything® Easy Gourmet Cookbook
Everything® Fondue Cookbook
Everything® **Fondue Party Book**
Everything® Gluten-Free Cookbook
Everything® Glycemic Index Cookbook
Everything® Grilling Cookbook

Everything® Healthy Meals in Minutes Cookbook
Everything® Holiday Cookbook
Everything® Indian Cookbook
Everything® Italian Cookbook
Everything® Low-Carb Cookbook
Everything® Low-Fat High-Flavor Cookbook
Everything® Low-Salt Cookbook
Everything® Meals for a Month Cookbook
Everything® Mediterranean Cookbook
Everything® Mexican Cookbook
Everything® One-Pot Cookbook
Everything® **Quick and Easy 30-Minute, 5-Ingredient Cookbook**
Everything® Quick Meals Cookbook
Everything® Slow Cooker Cookbook
Everything® Slow Cooking for a Crowd Cookbook
Everything® Soup Cookbook
Everything® Tex-Mex Cookbook
Everything® Thai Cookbook
Everything® Vegetarian Cookbook
Everything® Wild Game Cookbook
Everything® Wine Book, 2nd Ed.

GAMES

Everything® 15-Minute Sudoku Book, $9.95
Everything® 30-Minute Sudoku Book, $9.95
Everything® Blackjack Strategy Book
Everything® Brain Strain Book, $9.95
Everything® Bridge Book
Everything® Card Games Book
Everything® Card Tricks Book, $9.95
Everything® Casino Gambling Book, 2nd Ed.
Everything® Chess Basics Book
Everything® Craps Strategy Book
Everything® Crossword and Puzzle Book
Everything® Crossword Challenge Book
Everything® Cryptograms Book, $9.95
Everything® Easy Crosswords Book
Everything® Easy Kakuro Book, $9.95
Everything® Games Book, 2nd Ed.
Everything® Giant Sudoku Book, $9.95
Everything® Kakuro Challenge Book, $9.95
Everything® **Large-Print Crossword Challenge Book**
Everything® Large-Print Crosswords Book
Everything® Lateral Thinking Puzzles Book, $9.95
Everything® **Mazes Book**

Everything® Pencil Puzzles Book, $9.95
Everything® Poker Strategy Book
Everything® Pool & Billiards Book
Everything® Test Your IQ Book, $9.95
Everything® Texas Hold 'Em Book, $9.95
Everything® Travel Crosswords Book, $9.95
Everything® Word Games Challenge Book
Everything® Word Search Book

HEALTH

Everything® Alzheimer's Book
Everything® Diabetes Book
Everything® Health Guide to Adult Bipolar Disorder
Everything® Health Guide to Controlling Anxiety
Everything® Health Guide to Fibromyalgia
Everything® **Health Guide to Thyroid Disease**
Everything® Hypnosis Book
Everything® Low Cholesterol Book
Everything® Massage Book
Everything® Menopause Book
Everything® Nutrition Book
Everything® Reflexology Book
Everything® Stress Management Book

HISTORY

Everything® American Government Book
Everything® American History Book
Everything® Civil War Book
Everything® Freemasons Book
Everything® Irish History & Heritage Book
Everything® Middle East Book

HOBBIES

Everything® Candlemaking Book
Everything® Cartooning Book
Everything® **Coin Collecting Book**
Everything® Drawing Book
Everything® Family Tree Book, 2nd Ed.
Everything® Knitting Book
Everything® Knots Book
Everything® Photography Book
Everything® Quilting Book
Everything® Scrapbooking Book
Everything® Sewing Book
Everything® Woodworking Book

Bolded titles are new additions to the series.
All Everything® books are priced at $12.95 or $14.95, unless otherwise stated. Prices subject to change without notice.

HOME IMPROVEMENT

Everything® Feng Shui Book
Everything® Feng Shui Decluttering Book, $9.95
Everything® Fix-It Book
Everything® Home Decorating Book
Everything® Home Storage Solutions Book
Everything® Homebuilding Book
Everything® Lawn Care Book
Everything® Organize Your Home Book

KIDS' BOOKS

All titles are $7.95

Everything® Kids' Animal Puzzle & Activity Book
Everything® Kids' Baseball Book, 4th Ed.
Everything® Kids' Bible Trivia Book
Everything® Kids' Bugs Book
Everything® Kids' Cars and Trucks Puzzle & Activity Book
Everything® Kids' Christmas Puzzle & Activity Book
Everything® Kids' Cookbook
Everything® Kids' Crazy Puzzles Book
Everything® Kids' Dinosaurs Book
Everything® Kids' First Spanish Puzzle and Activity Book
Everything® Kids' Gross Hidden Pictures Book
Everything® Kids' Gross Jokes Book
Everything® Kids' Gross Mazes Book
Everything® Kids' Gross Puzzle and Activity Book
Everything® Kids' Halloween Puzzle & Activity Book
Everything® Kids' Hidden Pictures Book
Everything® Kids' Horses Book
Everything® Kids' Joke Book
Everything® Kids' Knock Knock Book
Everything® Kids' Learning Spanish Book
Everything® Kids' Math Puzzles Book
Everything® Kids' Mazes Book
Everything® Kids' Money Book
Everything® Kids' Nature Book
Everything® Kids' Pirates Puzzle and Activity Book
Everything® Kids' Princess Puzzle and Activity Book
Everything® Kids' Puzzle Book
Everything® Kids' Riddles & Brain Teasers Book
Everything® Kids' Science Experiments Book
Everything® Kids' Sharks Book
Everything® Kids' Soccer Book
Everything® Kids' Travel Activity Book

KIDS' STORY BOOKS

Everything® Fairy Tales Book

LANGUAGE

Everything® Conversational Chinese Book with CD, $19.95
Everything® Conversational Japanese Book with CD, $19.95
Everything® French Grammar Book
Everything® French Phrase Book, $9.95
Everything® French Verb Book, $9.95
Everything® German Practice Book with CD, $19.95
Everything® Inglés Book
Everything® Learning French Book
Everything® Learning German Book
Everything® Learning Italian Book
Everything® Learning Latin Book
Everything® Learning Spanish Book
Everything® Russian Practice Book with CD, $19.95
Everything® Sign Language Book
Everything® Spanish Grammar Book
Everything® Spanish Phrase Book, $9.95
Everything® Spanish Practice Book with CD, $19.95
Everything® Spanish Verb Book, $9.95

MUSIC

Everything® Drums Book with CD, $19.95
Everything® Guitar Book
Everything® Guitar Chords Book with CD, $19.95
Everything® Home Recording Book
Everything® Music Theory Book with CD, $19.95
Everything® Reading Music Book with CD, $19.95
Everything® Rock & Blues Guitar Book (with CD), $19.95
Everything® Songwriting Book

NEW AGE

Everything® Astrology Book, 2nd Ed.
Everything® Birthday Personology Book
Everything® Dreams Book, 2nd Ed.
Everything® Love Signs Book, $9.95
Everything® Numerology Book
Everything® Paganism Book
Everything® Palmistry Book
Everything® Psychic Book
Everything® Reiki Book
Everything® Sex Signs Book, $9.95
Everything® Tarot Book, 2nd Ed.
Everything® Wicca and Witchcraft Book

PARENTING

Everything® Baby Names Book, 2nd Ed.
Everything® Baby Shower Book
Everything® Baby's First Food Book
Everything® Baby's First Year Book
Everything® Birthing Book
Everything® Breastfeeding Book
Everything® Father-to-Be Book
Everything® Father's First Year Book
Everything® Get Ready for Baby Book
Everything® Get Your Baby to Sleep Book, $9.95
Everything® Getting Pregnant Book
Everything® Guide to Raising a One-Year-Old
Everything® Guide to Raising a Two-Year-Old
Everything® Homeschooling Book
Everything® Mother's First Year Book
Everything® Parent's Guide to Children and Divorce
Everything® Parent's Guide to Children with ADD/ADHD
Everything® Parent's Guide to Children with Asperger's Syndrome
Everything® Parent's Guide to Children with Autism
Everything® Parent's Guide to Children with Bipolar Disorder
Everything® Parent's Guide to Children with Dyslexia
Everything® Parent's Guide to Positive Discipline
Everything® Parent's Guide to Raising a Successful Child
Everything® Parent's Guide to Raising Boys
Everything® Parent's Guide to Raising Siblings
Everything® Parent's Guide to Sensory Integration Disorder
Everything® Parent's Guide to Tantrums
Everything® Parent's Guide to the Overweight Child
Everything® Parent's Guide to the Strong-Willed Child
Everything® Parenting a Teenager Book
Everything® Potty Training Book, $9.95
Everything® Pregnancy Book, 2nd Ed.
Everything® Pregnancy Fitness Book
Everything® Pregnancy Nutrition Book
Everything® Pregnancy Organizer, 2nd Ed., $16.95
Everything® Toddler Activities Book
Everything® Toddler Book
Everything® Tween Book
Everything® Twins, Triplets, and More Book

PETS

Everything® Aquarium Book
Everything® Boxer Book
Everything® Cat Book, 2nd Ed.
Everything® Chihuahua Book
Everything® Dachshund Book
Everything® Dog Book
Everything® Dog Health Book
Everything® Dog Owner's Organizer, $16.95
Everything® Dog Training and Tricks Book
Everything® German Shepherd Book
Everything® Golden Retriever Book
Everything® Horse Book
Everything® Horse Care Book
Everything® Horseback Riding Book
Everything® Labrador Retriever Book
Everything® Poodle Book
Everything® Pug Book
Everything® Puppy Book
Everything® Rottweiler Book
Everything® Small Dogs Book
Everything® Tropical Fish Book
Everything® Yorkshire Terrier Book

REFERENCE

Everything® Blogging Book
Everything® Build Your Vocabulary Book
Everything® Car Care Book
Everything® Classical Mythology Book
Everything® Da Vinci Book
Everything® Divorce Book
Everything® Einstein Book
Everything® Etiquette Book, 2nd Ed.
Everything® Inventions and Patents Book
Everything® Mafia Book
Everything® Philosophy Book
Everything® Psychology Book
Everything® Shakespeare Book

RELIGION

Everything® Angels Book
Everything® Bible Book
Everything® Buddhism Book
Everything® Catholicism Book
Everything® Christianity Book
Everything® History of the Bible Book
Everything® Jesus Book
Everything® Jewish History & Heritage Book
Everything® Judaism Book
Everything® Kabbalah Book
Everything® Koran Book
Everything® Mary Book

Everything® Mary Magdalene Book
Everything® Prayer Book
Everything® Saints Book
Everything® Torah Book
Everything® Understanding Islam Book
Everything® World's Religions Book
Everything® Zen Book

SCHOOL & CAREERS

Everything® Alternative Careers Book
Everything® Career Tests Book
Everything® College Major Test Book
Everything® College Survival Book, 2nd Ed.
Everything® Cover Letter Book, 2nd Ed.
Everything® Filmmaking Book
Everything® Get-a-Job Book
Everything® Guide to Being a Paralegal
Everything® Guide to Being a Real Estate Agent
Everything® Guide to Being a Sales Rep
Everything® Guide to Careers in Health Care
Everything® Guide to Careers in Law Enforcement
Everything® Guide to Government Jobs
Everything® Guide to Starting and Running a Restaurant
Everything® Job Interview Book
Everything® New Nurse Book
Everything® New Teacher Book
Everything® Paying for College Book
Everything® Practice Interview Book
Everything® Resume Book, 2nd Ed.
Everything® Study Book

SELF-HELP

Everything® Dating Book, 2nd Ed.
Everything® Great Sex Book
Everything® Kama Sutra Book
Everything® Self-Esteem Book

SPORTS & FITNESS

Everything® Easy Fitness Book
Everything® Fishing Book
Everything® Golf Instruction Book
Everything® Pilates Book
Everything® Running Book
Everything® Weight Training Book
Everything® Yoga Book

TRAVEL

Everything® Family Guide to Cruise Vacations
Everything® Family Guide to Hawaii

Everything® Family Guide to Las Vegas, 2nd Ed.
Everything® Family Guide to Mexico
Everything® Family Guide to New York City, 2nd Ed.
Everything® Family Guide to RV Travel & Campgrounds
Everything® Family Guide to the Caribbean
Everything® Family Guide to the Walt Disney World Resort®, Universal Studios®, and Greater Orlando, 4th Ed.
Everything® Family Guide to Timeshares
Everything® Family Guide to Washington D.C., 2nd Ed.
Everything® Guide to New England

WEDDINGS

Everything® Bachelorette Party Book, $9.95
Everything® Bridesmaid Book, $9.95
Everything® Destination Wedding Book
Everything® Elopement Book, $9.95
Everything® Father of the Bride Book, $9.95
Everything® Groom Book, $9.95
Everything® Mother of the Bride Book, $9.95
Everything® Outdoor Wedding Book
Everything® Wedding Book, 3rd Ed.
Everything® Wedding Checklist, $9.95
Everything® Wedding Etiquette Book, $9.95
Everything® Wedding Organizer, 2nd Ed., $16.95
Everything® Wedding Shower Book, $9.95
Everything® Wedding Vows Book, $9.95
Everything® Wedding Workout Book
Everything® Weddings on a Budget Book, $9.95

WRITING

Everything® Creative Writing Book
Everything® Get Published Book, 2nd Ed.
Everything® Grammar and Style Book
Everything® Guide to Writing a Book Proposal
Everything® Guide to Writing a Novel
Everything® Guide to Writing Children's Books
Everything® Guide to Writing Research Papers
Everything® Screenwriting Book
Everything® Writing Poetry Book
Everything® Writing Well Book